Gill Wh...

health + happiness

How to Work Wonders
Your Guide to Workplace Wellness

Lots of love

Liggy

How to Work Wonders

Your Guide to Workplace Wellness

by

Liggy Webb

Grosvenor House
Publishing Limited

Liggy Webb is hereby identified as author of this
work in accordance with Section 77 of the Copyright, Designs
and Patents Act 1988

Graphic Designer - Kate Tuck
Copy Editor - Lawrence McIlhoney
Cartoons - Richard Duszczak
Tel: +44 (0)1246 209034
Email: info@cartoonstudio.co.uk
Ordering Information
Individual orders and quantity sales (discounts available)
Mail to: info@thelearningarchitect.com
Tel: +44 (0)1242 700027

This book is published by
Grosvenor House Publishing Ltd
28-30 High Street, Guildford, Surrey, GU1 3HY.
www.grosvenorhousepublishing.co.uk

A CIP record for this book
is available from the British Library

ISBN 978-1-906645-91-5

Alternatively you can order from www.amazon.co.uk

**Please note, that this book cannot, nor is intended to,
replace the services of a qualified medical professional.**

This book is dedicated to my parents Robin and Ann
You are a constant source of
unconditional love, support and inspiration

Thankyou

Contents

Acknowledgements

First of all, I would like to thank Kate Tuck (Batman Rodney) without whose help and support I would not have been able to write this book. Thank you for your friendship, intelligence and fantastic sense of humour! What an amazing journey!

Lawrence McIlhoney, my Editor. You have the patience of a saint, the eye of an eagle and the wonderful thing about tiggers is that tiggers are wonderful things.

I would also like to acknowledge and thank the following people for their love and support:

Everyone who is part of *The Learning Architect*. You are an amazingly talented group of people.

All the members of *The Montpellier Writing Group* and in loving memory of Julie Savage.

Sara Pankhurst, *my soul sister*. For your belief, love, trust and a whole recycling bin of *little tartan diaries*.

Andy Veitch and Adrian Coubrough – My bookends. Thank you so much for *always* being there.

Melanie Lisney – For your wonderful wisdom and friendship.

George Richards – Thank you for everything and now for another carrot baton?

Aubrey Stuart – You just gotta make it happen baby!

Richard Duzczak for your super cartoons.

Kim, Maggi and Ruth at Grosvenor House Publishing for putting it all together.

And to all my wonderful family and friends who have helped me to *work wonders* through all my *probortunities*.

Thankyou.

Introduction

I don't like Mondays
tell me why?
I don't like Mondays.
I want to shoot
the whole day down.

— *Bob Geldof*

Monday Morning Blues

The words to this song, a number one hit for The Boomtown Rats in 1979, may resonate if you have (along with many others) a real aversion to Monday mornings. For some, it is the most challenging time of all to separate yourself from the warmth and comfort of your duvet and the morning you abuse the snooze on your alarm clock repeatedly, in a vain attempt to postpone the inevitable start of yet another dreaded week at work.

In fact, research suggests that more heart attacks occur on a Monday morning than any other day of the week. An explanation for this could be that many people are free of the mental and physical burdens of work on a Sunday and experience a more stressful change from weekend leisure to work activities.

Bob Geldof wrote the lyrics to *I don't like Mondays* after reading a telex report at Georgia State

University on the shooting spree of 16-year-old Brenda Ann Spencer who fired at children playing in a school playground across the street from her home in California. She killed two adults and injured eight children and one police officer. Spencer showed no remorse for her crime and her full explanation for her actions was "I don't like Mondays; this livens up the day" - clearly an extreme reaction to what is commonly known as 'Monday morning blues'.

Interestingly enough, there is a scientific explanation behind those morning blues. Our internal clocks naturally operate on a day that is longer than 24 hours. By the time Monday rolls around each week, we've built up a sleep deficit of at least an hour. This, combined with common clichés like "Thank God it's Friday", can easily condition your mind to react in a negative way to the beginning of the working week.

So, can you imagine waking up on a Monday morning, not wanting to shoot the whole day down and actually viewing it as the beginning of a wonderful new week? Well, the great news is that you can - this book is about helping you to develop a healthy and positive attitude and approach to work and indeed everything that you do in your life!

Working in the 21st Century

Many of us spend the biggest proportion of our lives at work and with our work colleagues, in some cases more time than we spend at home and with our friends and relatives.

Work is fast becoming the way in which we define ourselves. It is now answering some of the traditional questions: "Who am I?" and "How do I find meaning and purpose?" Work is no longer just about economics; it's about identity. About fifty years ago, people had many sources of identity: religion, class, nationality, political affiliation, family roots, geographical and cultural origins and more. Today, many of these, if not all, have been superseded by work.

When you meet someone at a party, what's one of the first questions that you are typically asked? "So, what do you *do* then."

Work is where we get to employ most of our talents. It's where we experience some of our greatest triumphs and failures. It's also the basis for our standard of living. All of this means that, when work is not working for us, we become unproductive and unfulfilled.

Being unhappy at work can make you sick and being happy at work can make you healthier. This sounds like an unlikely claim at first, but it's perfectly true.

Lancaster University and Manchester Business School performed a study in 2005 involving 250,000 employees which found that low happiness at work is a risk factor for mental health problems, including emotional burn-out, low self-esteem, anxiety and depression. The report warned that just a small drop in job satisfaction could lead to burnout of *considerable clinical importance*.

Mental stress symptoms like the ones found in the study also increase the risk of physical health issues including ulcers, heart problems and a weakened immune system.

In today's workplace, wellness is becoming an increasingly topical issue. With terms like *stress-related illness* and *burnout* becoming household words, many organisations are increasingly looking for ways to reduce stress and absenteeism. With environmental, equality and diversity policies now in place, it seems highly likely that a mandatory *Workplace Wellness policy* will be next on the agenda.

Having spent the past few years conducting research across a wide range of organisations both in the UK and internationally, I am heartened to see some very responsible actions and transformations taking place. There are some excellent examples of organisations that actively promote healthy practices and raise awareness by providing programmes within the workplace to encourage healthier behaviours.

It is, nevertheless, important to be realistic about the extent to which organisations can support individuals and a sense of personal responsibility is essential. Work is what YOU make it and it is your attitude and approach that will have the most significant effect.

Work - Life Balance

Looking after people in the workplace is becoming an increasingly important issue and an appreciation for *Work-Life Balance* is a phrase that has been bandied about since the 1970s. Over the past thirty years, there has been a substantial increase in workload which is felt to be due, in part, to the use of information technology and to an intense, competitive work environment.

Long-term loyalty and a sense of corporate community have been eroded by a performance culture that expects more and more from employees yet offers little support in return.

Many experts forecasted that technology would eliminate most household chores and provide people with much more time to enjoy leisure activities. Unfortunately, many have decided to ignore this option, *being egged on* by a consumerist culture and a political agenda that has elevated the work ethic to unprecedented heights.

An alarming amount of absenteeism in the workplace is now stress-related and it is clear that problems caused by stress have become a major concern to both employers and employees. Symptoms are manifested both physiologically and psychologically. Persistent stress can result in a range of problems, including frequent headaches, stiff muscles and backache. It can also result in irritability, insecurity, exhaustion and difficulty concentrating.

Stress can also lead to eating disorders, increased smoking, excessive caffeine and increased alcohol consumption. These, in turn, will perpetuate depression and mental illness, so the vicious cycle of negativity continues.

The impact of absenteeism on the economy is colossal. However, another important area to consider is that of *presenteeism*. In contrast to absenteeism, presenteeism is when employees come to work in spite of illness which can have similar negative repercussions on business performance. A depressed economic climate and the threat of redundancy can put people under considerable pressure to come into work. However, work performance is impaired, expensive mistakes are made and this can have serious repercussions.

So what is the answer? Well, realistically there is no magic formula; however, there are certainly measures that can be taken to address some of the health issues that occur. Learning to manage personal stress can help considerably, and a better understanding of what we can do to help ourselves is extremely important.

Organisations that help raise awareness for healthier working practices are taking responsibility and finding that they are being rewarded by a reduction in absenteeism, better morale, long-term loyalty and a sense of corporate community. These factors clearly contribute to a far happier and more productive workplace.

Why Work Wonders?

I was compelled to write this book for a variety of reasons, both professionally and personally. In my capacity as a learning and development professional it has become increasingly clear to me that, in order to implement sustainable learning, individuals need to be fully receptive and engaged. Therefore, if the work environment and the physical and mental wellness of employees are not conducive to a healthy "can do" and "want to do" attitude, the potential and channel for real learning and development is inhibited.

Another key motivator is a little more personal, yet very relative to the work environment. Depression affects a staggering 120 million people worldwide and is a very real medical condition. It is estimated that, by 2020, depression will be one of the leading causes of disability and ill health. High levels of stress in the work place can be a dangerous trigger and it is critical that individuals and organisations adopt strategies to mitigate the risk of exacerbating the situation. Having personally experienced depression, I am fully empathetic and aware of how individuals can struggle at work when experiencing episodes of the illness.

In retrospect, my first hand experience has taught me many valuable lessons. I feel somewhat enlightened and enthused by what I have learnt and wanted to share this and help others to manage personal stress and depression, as not only is it debilitating, but also highly damaging with long term health implications.

While some organisations take a more proactive approach to looking after the wellness of their people, individuals also need to be prepared to take more responsibility for themselves. *How to Work Wonders* is about raising awareness of what we can do to help ourselves. It is not about massive transformations or an unrealistic metamorphosis. It is about an appreciation of the little things that we can do in our everyday lives to improve and balance our overall health. By tackling the little things, which may seem insignificant in isolation, we can stop these mounting up until they become something that we cannot cope with.

So what will this book help you to do?

- Develop a positive approach to work and life.
- Benefit from exercise and healthy eating.
- Manage your emotions and stress levels.
- Communicate more positively and effectively.
- Improve your working environment.
- Set personal action plans and achieve result.

For this book to really help, you will need to address some of your existing habits and cultivate new ones. This is not always easy to do and, personally, I find that working on the 80/20 rule is by far the best approach. Many attempts to give up bad habits fail because once we fall off track, we beat ourselves up and console ourselves, perversely, by falling back into the bad habit that we are trying to move away from. So, cutting yourself a bit of slack is a far more realistic approach and makes "getting it right 80% of the time" much more achievable.

One of my key observations is that *Workplace Wellness* is about taking a holistic approach. It is not really enough to be physically fit and healthy in isolation of other elements that affect you. These involve your attitude to your work, your communication skills, how you manage personal stress, improvements that you can contribute to your work environment and being aware of how you can set goals and take personal action.

The following enablers will all be explored in the subsequent chapters of this book and summarised with useful and practical *How to Work Wonders* tips. Each part plays an equally valuable role in the holistic pursuit of Workplace Wellness.

- Attitude
- Exercise & Nutrition
- Communication
- Stress Management
- Environment
- Goal Setting

How to Work Wonders is a guide that will offer you information and advice on how you can make the most of your own mental, physical and environmental health at work. Please note, that this book cannot, nor is intended to, replace the services of a qualified medical professional.

Happy reading and I hope that this book works wonders for you!

> *Your work is to discover your work and then with all your heart to give yourself to it. That's the mark of a true professional.*
> —*Buddha*

CHAPTER ONE - ATTITUDE

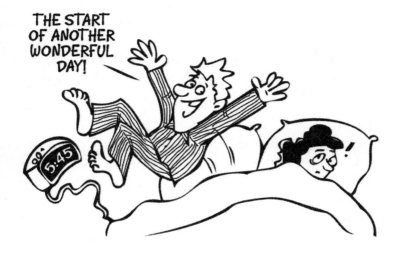

Your attitude, not your aptitude, will determine your altitude

Zig Ziglar

The term *Positive Mental Attitude* has almost become a bit of a cliché. Every book on success or self-improvement starts with a sharp focus on cultivating energy, enthusiasm and optimism in all areas of your life and, in my view, quite rightly so. Positive thinking is the key to happiness and health and pretty much dictates the way we go about our work and live our lives in general.

A positive attitude is not about a magical mystical mindset possessed by the lucky few. It is something that *everyone* is capable of achieving and is simply an inclination or leaning toward the positive aspects of any given situation. Thinking positively is not about putting your head in the sand; nor is it about being unrealistic. A positive attitude recognises the negative aspects of a situation, however chooses to focus instead on the hope and opportunity available. This releases you from getting locked in a paralysing loop of bad feeling and allows you to move quickly to take action and solve difficulties.

Positive thinking and optimism are now known to be a root cause of many life benefits. The relatively new science of *Psychoneuroimmunology* looks at how our mind can influence our immune system. The theory is that you will live longer and be healthier and happier by cultivating a positive attitude toward life. In addition, you're more likely to be successful, maintain better relationships and have a beneficial influence on those around you.

Your mental approach to life is a combination of your thoughts, emotions and beliefs. Becoming aware of your emotions, identifying and analysing your thoughts and understanding your beliefs is key to really being able to tackle how you deal with what comes your way.

It is not necessarily what happens to you in life; it is how you react to it.

The most basic indicators of your positivity or negativity are your emotions, which are essentially a mental state that arises spontaneously rather than through conscious effort, and are often accompanied by physiological changes.

Your emotions can have a very strong impact on how you behave and react. Emotional Intelligence (EQ) is a relatively recent behavioural model, rising to prominence with Daniel Goleman's 1995 book called *Emotional Intelligence*. It is a fascinating area and well worth reading up on to help you to become more emotionally aware. The essential premise of Emotional Intelligence is that, in order to be successful, you require the awareness, control and management of your own emotions and recognise and understand the emotions of those around you.

It is important also to be aware that you feed your emotions with your thoughts. Here is an analogy to illustrate this concept that conjures up a wonderful visual image:

Imagine you are hosting a dinner party for all your emotions and they are sitting around the dinner table hungrily waiting to be fed. All the usual suspects are there like fear, anger, jealousy, happiness, optimism, joy and an assortment of the good, the bad and the downright ugly. You are there as the host of the dinner party and you can choose which emotion you want to feed.

In the same way, by choosing what you think, you can starve the negative emotions and feed up and boost the health of the positive ones. You are in fact the nutritionist of your soul. What a great concept!

It also helps to remember that, at the bedrock of your thoughts and emotions are your values and beliefs, deep rooted ideas that are a result of all your life experiences. These are your life attitudes and they colour and shape your perception of the world. Whereas thoughts are relative, beliefs tend to feel completely true, undeniable and resolute. Negative beliefs, however, can undermine your joy in life, so it is well worth addressing any negative beliefs and looking to change them for a positive alternative.

Being consciously aware of your thoughts, feelings and beliefs can be a very useful exercise and the ability to challenge our thoughts can be a positive step in helping us to identify negative behaviours and ultimately discover positive solutions to problems and opportunities.

I was delighted to find that a new word has been introduced into our vocabulary called *Probortunity*. This inclusive word combines *problem* and *opportunity* to describe something you want to improve and change for the better. Positive thinking is a habit anyone can adopt with some practice, irrespective of their background, education and experience.

Understanding Habits

For you to really benefit from this book, it is important that you are prepared to make some changes, break a few bad habits and embrace a few new ones. So, first of all, understanding habits and how they form is going to be very useful.

> *Habits are at first cobwebs, and then they become cables*
>
> —*Spanish Proverb*

The human brain is a magnificent machine and consists of billions of nerve cells with innumerable extensions. This interlacing of nerve fibres and their junctions allows a nerve impulse to follow a number of routes known as *neural pathways*. When you learn something new, your brain makes connections that create new pathways for activity. Setting up neural pathways is actually quite simple. If a newly-learned behaviour is repeated enough times, it eventually gets programmed into the subconscious mind; that behaviour becomes automatic and we no longer have to think about doing it, because we respond automatically. This, simply put, is a habit.

Have you ever arrived at home or work with no memory of how you got there? When you started on your journey, you thought about the first few steps on that familiar path, but somewhere along the way, your brain moved onto more interesting topics, and the next thing you knew, you'd arrived. This is the essence of habits: once you start on a familiar series of actions, you stop thinking about them and you are able to complete them without conscious thought or attention.

Cache memory in a computer is another good analogy. The computer stores commonly-used actions where it can access and process them faster. The brain does the same thing. This can work in both a positive and negative way as it can free up our minds from dull or repetitive tasks, although it also makes it difficult to stop once we've started.

Over 90% of our daily routine is comprised of various habits that create our behaviours. What separates the positive and negative people is that the positive people have habits and behaviours that are conducive to success, while the negative people have ones that facilitate failure in their lives. Remember: you control your habits - they do not control you. Your life is the culmination of all the daily behaviours that you have.

You are where you are right now because of the behaviours that you have adopted in the past.

It is important to identify which habits in your life lead to negative consequences and which lead to positive rewards. The difficulty in this sometimes has to do with instant gratification. If you change your habits, on occasions you're not going to see an immediate effect. It is for this reason that people struggle with diets or can't stop drinking, smoking, or spending money because they can't control the instant gratification that is delivered.

Experts in hypnosis and NLP (Neuro-Linguistic Programming – which is the art and science of personal excellence) believe that it takes around 21 to 28 days to form the basis of a new habit or behaviour. The time it takes to replace an old one is inconclusive because it depends entirely on the person and how long they have *owned* it.

Think of behaviour as a tree. One that is fairly new is like a young tree with short roots that you can pull straight from the ground. A behaviour that you have owned for many years is like an adult tree that has long roots that extend far underground.

Human beings tend to take actions to either move them closer to pleasure or away from pain. With that in mind, analyse your bad habits and dig for the underlying factors involved with them. Why do you eat so much? Why do you drink so much? Why are you negative? Behind all of these habits and behaviours lies a reason. Changing a bad behaviour without addressing the root cause of the problem will only lead to a regression.

As with any newly learned behaviour, you may well experience some internal resistance for the first week or more. This is natural and it's not going to be easy, so you have to mentally prepare for this challenge ahead of time. After you survive this first week, you will find that your new habit and behaviour becomes easier and easier to do and soon you don't even have to think about doing it at all.

Stress is the primary cause of people reverting back to their old patterns of behaviour, so be wary of the level of stress in your life and know that a high amount can wipe away a new habit and make you revert back to your old ones.

How to Develop Good Habits

✓ Challenge yourself and believe that you can do it.
✓ Identify exactly the specific habit that you would like to change.
✓ Make a list of all the benefits of breaking or adopting the habit.
✓ Set yourself up for success by taking *immediate* action to change.
✓ Tell people around you what you are trying to do.
✓ Don't give up. Failure is only a reality when you stop trying.

✓ Keep a record of your progress and results.
✓ Make sure you keep it up even when you have succeeded.
✓ Be positive and open minded about change.

It is not the strongest of the species that survives, or the most intelligent, but rather the one most adaptable to change
—*Charles Darwin*

The Power of Positive Thinking

Years ago, my grandmother introduced me to a book called *The Power of Positive Thinking* by Norman Vincent Peale. Peale's works came under criticism from several mental health experts, one of whom directly said Peale was a conman and a fraud. His book, however, went on to become a phenomenal and inspiring best seller. One of my favourite quotes is: *"Change your thoughts and you change your world"*. So true, and another one that is worth contemplation is: *"Change yourself and your work will seem different"*.

Creating and maintaining a positive attitude is the most efficient and low-cost investment you can make in order to improve your life. A positive way of thinking is a habit that must be learned through repetition and conscious effort on your part.

Positive affirmations to condition your mind can be very useful. Saying things to yourself like:

*I am an optimistic, hopeful, positive thinking person.
I accept that bad things may happen in my life, but I
look for positive opportunities in the midst of anything
negative.*

A positive attitude is not *dependent* upon your
genetic composition even if you are pre-disposed to
negative thinking you can *learn* to move your thinking
to the positive side.

This depends upon how you *choose* to think.

We are faced with literally millions of challenging
situations throughout our personal and professional
lives. By accepting the reality that we will be faced
with many challenges, to which we must seek
solutions, it becomes obvious that creating and
maintaining a positive attitude can only help us. Our
problems remain the same size; it does not matter if
you react with bitterness or enthusiasm, and it
doesn't change the problem.

How to Think Positively

✓ Declare your intent to think positively.
✓ Write down your intention in strong, clear and
   direct language.
✓ Use positive affirmations to condition your mind.
✓ Read inspiring books and listen to audio tapes on
   the subject.
✓ At the end of each day, reflect on the positive
   aspects of the day.

✓ Become very aware of your thinking and internal voice.
✓ Before going to sleep, reflect upon what you're looking forward to the next day.
✓ Write down any concerns you have and challenge them with a positive outcome.

Are you a NAG carrier?

I have been lucky enough to work with and meet some highly successful and inspiring people. What sets them aside and makes them special is their ability to turn a potentially negative thought into a positive one. They are also acutely aware of their attitude and how it affects others around them. They take responsibility for their NAGs - Negative Attitude Germs!

Let me ask you a question. If you had a really bad cold or flu would you walk over to someone and sneeze in their face? Hopefully not!

So let me ask you another question. Have you ever had a bad day when someone or something has annoyed or upset you and you have felt the need to get it off your chest and tell someone else all about it? I am sure that we have all been guilty of that from time to time.

You are, in effect, spreading your NAGs - Negative Attitude Germs.

You may have noticed that when you are with someone who is suffering from a physical or emotional problem, you feel bad too. It's often described as *catching their emotion*. Researchers have observed this actually happening in real time in the brain, using an advanced MRI (Magnetic Resonance Imaging) machine. It shows the brain of Person A reflects activity in the same area as Person B when they are in close proximity.

The scientific term for this is *neural mirroring*. This does, therefore, point out the danger of hanging around negative, pessimistic people if you prefer to be positive and optimistic. You can "catch" their NAGs just by being in close proximity.

Another analogy I like to use is drains and radiators. Which are you?

Drains and Radiators

Some people you meet are like drains: negative, listless doom goblins and when we come into contact with them they drain us of energy. They like to tell you about negative news and when you ask them how they are they will respond with their shoulders slumped, eyelids drooped *"Well you know … I feel really … bad!"* and then they will give you a graphic blow by blow account of all their woes and feelings of impending doom!

Other people, however, are like radiators - full of warmth and vitality. We feel positively energised by them. They appear bright and radiant, look you in the eye and when you ask them how they are, they smile and tell you something positive. My mother is a great example of a radiator because no matter how she feels, she doesn't dump her negativity on to other people and remains positive and strong in the face of adversity. She talks constructively about overcoming problems and finding solutions. It is, as I have come to appreciate over the years, a much kinder and more responsible way to live.

Every year, I am invited to deliver motivational talks on P&O cruise ships on the subject of the mind-body link and how we can improve our overall wellbeing by being positive and goal-orientated. Last year, a gentleman came up to me afterwards, looked me straight in the eye with a big smile on his face and said "I thoroughly enjoyed your talk and agree with everything you say – how old do you think I am? Go on guess."

I looked at him, his smile, his demeanour, his posture and guessed at late sixties. He took me absolutely by surprise when he responded "I am eighty six and I'm a radiator because no matter how I feel, if anyone asks me how I am, I tell them I feel good and happy to be alive and then I tell myself the same thing and then I am!" What a fantastic attitude and a glowing example of radiator behaviour.

How to be a Radiator

✓ Walk tall irrespective of your height.
✓ Look people in the eyes when you talk to them.
✓ Take pride in your appearance.

✓ Empathise with other people.
✓ Be self-aware and emotionally intelligent.
✓ See the glass half full, NOT half empty.
✓ Develop a positive vocabulary.
✓ Look for the opportunity, not the obstacle.
✓ Make the most of every day.

Your Most Valuable Asset

Your brain is your most valuable asset when it comes to attitude. It is the hardware of your soul. How your brain works determines how happy you are, how capable you feel, how you interact with others.

Until recently, scientists could only speculate about the brain's role in defining our personalities and behaviours. There were not the advanced tools that we have now to look at the functioning of the brain and false assumptions were made about its impact on our lives. With the advent of sophisticated brain-imaging techniques, the brain's role in behaviour is being explored and examined at a phenomenal pace and we are learning more each day.

I think it is such an exciting and fascinating time to be around as the mysteries of the mind are unfolding and we are learning more and more about the incredible instrument that we have in our possession. To try to explain the function of the human brain would be a book in itself; however, there is one part of your brain that plays a vital part in your ability to achieve positive outcomes and influence your way of thinking. This is known as your Reticular Activating System.

Reticular Activating System

Your Reticular Activating System (RAS) is a wonderfully evolved part of your brain that is a filter between your conscious mind and your subconscious mind. It takes instructions from your conscious mind and passes them on to your subconscious.

For example, suppose I invited you all now to come and join me for a weekend in my home town of Cheltenham in the heart of the Cotswolds. We all go out together and do the same things, go for a long walk in the hills, lunch somewhere scenic, a bit of shopping, a movie maybe and then we all congregate at my favourite restaurant, *The Daffodil*, and compare our weekend. After discussion, we would inevitably find that, despite the fact that we shared the experience together, we would all have had different experiences simply because our RAS would have filtered different things.

So why does it do this? We are literally bombarded with sensory images, sounds and goings on all day long. Just imagine what your life would be like if you were aware of every single one of them - it would be mental bedlam! The RAS consists of a bundle of densely packed nerve cells located in the central core of the brainstem. Roughly the size of a little finger, the RAS runs from the top of the spinal cord into the middle of the brain. This area of tightly packed nerve fibres and cells contain nearly 70% of your brain's nerve cells.

The RAS acts as the executive secretary for your conscious mind. It is the chief gatekeeper to screen or filter the type of information that will be allowed to get through. Everything else is filtered out. You simply don't pay attention to those other "messages". Like restaurant noise when you are engrossed in a meaningful conversation, you screen it out.

There are some interesting points about your reticular activating system that make it an essential tool for achieving goals.

First of all you can deliberately programme the reticular activating system by choosing your exact messages, goals, affirmations, or visualisations. Napoleon Hill, the famous American author, said that we can achieve any realistic goal if we keep on thinking of that goal and stop thinking any negative thoughts about it.

What the mind of man can conceive and believe, it can achieve.

Of course, if we keep thinking that we can't achieve a goal; our subconscious will help us to not achieve it. Secondly, your reticular activating system cannot distinguish between real events and 'synthetic' reality. In other words, it tends to believe whatever message you give it.

What we need to do is to create a very specific picture of our desired outcome in our conscious mind. The RAS will then pass this on to our subconscious - which will then help us achieve what we are positively focused on. It does this by bringing to our attention all the relevant information which otherwise might have remained as background noise.

Something else to consider is the little voice inside your head, the one that chatters away to you all day long telling you all the things that you can do and what you can't do, what you like, what you don't like. We feed our RAS with thoughts and internal self-talk. Remember you control your RAS, it doesn't control you - so the more attention you pay to what you are feeding it, the more chance you will have to develop that all important positive attitude.

Have you got NITs?

What I mean by this is: have you got *Negative Inhibiting Thoughts* plaguing your head? Making your mind itch? We are at times our own worst enemy and the biggest crime that we commit towards our self is the inhibitors and excuses we create. Here are a few typical examples of excuses.

- The classic: "I can't".
- The ultimate cork in the works: "Yes but ...".
- "I haven't had the right upbringing".
- "I haven't had the right education".
- "I have never been any good at that".
- "The last time I tried that it didn't work".

Do you recognise any of these familiar excuses? Perhaps you do. However, the only person ultimately that you are making excuses to is yourself and stopping yourself from fully exploring your own potential.

Some behavioural psychologists believe that we are like acorns and inside each tiny acorn there is the potential to grow a beautiful oak tree. Many people, who don't break out of their acorn shell, will never have the opportunity to spread their branches and feel the splendour of growth and altitude. That is why Abraham Maslow assigns only 1% of the population to the pinnacle of self-actualisation, the ultimate quest to become the best you can be.

Some people practically have a Ph.D. in excuse making; however I am sure we all fall into the excuse trap occasionally, after all we are only human. Essentially, we are driven by two key motivators: fear and desire. If fear overrides desire, we will make excuses to protect and defend ourselves.

Excuses help us to remain in our comfort zone and negate responsibility, and it is responsibility that separates man from the rest of the animal kingdom. Unlike other animals, we are responsible not for what we have, but for what we could have; not for what we are, but for what we could become. If we are to take credit for our successes, we must assume responsibility for our failures. Excuses are harmful because they prevent us from succeeding. When we make excuses and repeat them often enough, they become a belief. The belief then becomes a self-fulfilling prophecy.

Just look at Thomas Edison, one of the most prolific inventors in history; how many attempts did he have trying to invent the light bulb? As the history books reveal over 10,000 attempts! We would certainly have been left in the dark if he had stopped because he had NITs!

How to Get Rid of Your NITs!

✓ Realise that your success or failure depends on you.
✓ Resolve to start accepting responsibility today.
✓ Don't find an excuse, find a way.
✓ Stop and examine your progress.
✓ Compare where you are now with where you would like to be.
✓ Make plans and take action.
✓ Listen to yourself and what is important to you.
✓ Don't let other people's negativity influence you.
✓ When you make a mistake, accept responsibility; learn from it.

The old dogma that an adult human brain is fixed and that you can't teach an old dog new tricks is wrong. The brain is amazingly flexible, changing in response constantly to experience and thought. You are never too old for personal growth.

Take Responsibility

The antidote for negativity is that you accept complete responsibility for your situation. The very act of taking responsibility short-circuits and cancels out any negative emotion that you may trigger. By embracing responsibility, we reap many rewards. The successes brought by this attitude act as a foundation for self-respect, pride and confidence. Responsibility breeds competence and power. By living up to our promises and obligations, we win the trust of others. Once we are seen as trustworthy, people will willingly work with us for our mutual gain. Making excuses can put the brakes on our progress, while accepting responsibility can lead us to succeed.

It is easy to blame others or circumstances for everything in our lives – past, present or future. It lets us off the hook to some degree. However, ultimately it doesn't help us because we become a prisoner of circumstance and allow everything and everyone around us to dictate our world.

As Eleanor Roosevelt so wisely proclaimed, "No-one can make you feel inferior without your consent". Have you ever heard yourself in an argument say "This is how YOU made me feel"? However the truth of the matter is that no one can make you feel anything – that is ultimately your choice – you choose how you feel.

Personally, I find the concept of personal responsibility very exciting because it provides you with the opportunity to make choices. We can choose how we want to react to everything.

So the next time something goes wrong, challenge whether you are looking for something or someone to blame and if you make a mistake say sorry and get busy rectifying the situation.

To keep your mind positive, refuse to criticise, complain about or condemn someone else. Complaining about someone else for something they have done or not done will only trigger feelings of negativity and anger in yourself. And then you are the one that suffers. Your negativity doesn't affect the other person at all. Being angry with someone is allowing them to control your emotions and often the entire quality of your life, long distance.

Once you take the decision to take complete responsibility for your own life and everything that happens to you, you can turn confidently to your work and your life and become *The ruler of your fate and the Master of your Soul.*

Self-Esteem

People who have high self-esteem tend to be positive thinkers. It seems to go with the territory. It follows that, if you use positive thinking to enhance your core beliefs, your self-esteem will soar.

If you were supporting someone with low self-esteem you wouldn't criticise or put them down. However, it's amazing how much of a hard time we can give ourselves, constantly beating ourselves up for the slightest mistake. Treating yourself how you would instinctively behave towards a friend is a much kinder way to behave towards yourself and far more positive.

Remember: for every mistake that you make, another valuable lesson you learn. So you are building your pot of wisdom. Working on your own self-confidence is key. There is a fine line between arrogance and confidence and it is important to be honest with yourself and seek feedback from others. It is also important, however, that you don't rely on others to *big you up* and make you feel better.

It is important that you learn how to recognise and congratulate yourself when you have done something well. If you rely on others or become so preoccupied with others' opinions of you, it can create insecurity and paranoia.

There is a wonderful poem called *Desiderata* written by Max Ehrmann. It is a masterpiece and makes a wonderful creed for life. This extract sums up what happens if you become too preoccupied with *other people:*

If you compare yourself with others,
you may become vain or bitter,
for always there will be greater and lesser persons
than yourself.
Enjoy your achievements as well as your plans.
Keep interested in your own career, however humble;
it is a real possession in the changing fortunes of time.

Imagine having no one to compare yourself with except yourself. What a sense of relief this would bring. We wouldn't have to beat ourselves up about not performing as well as our colleagues at work.

We wouldn't have to worry about not looking like the alpha male or female with the smartest mind, the most important job role and the biggest pay packet. We wouldn't have to worry about our bodies not being the youngest, most beautiful and most sexy.

All we would have to think is: did I do this activity better than I did it last week? Have I moved forward in my own definition of *success*? Am I feeling peaceful, doing my best for my health? Do I have an attractive mind and healthy interactions with other people?

Many of us would never admit to making comparisons with other people – to do so implies jealousy and small-mindedness. However, everyone has undoubtedly taken a measure of themselves at some point by reference to someone else – even if only subconsciously. We may have moved on from caveman (or rather cave people!), from times of comparing brute strength and hunting skills, but the *alpha caveman* has simply been replaced by the *alpha executive*. Now, our strengths are measured by whether we can outsmart colleagues, our status amongst peers and the cars we drive. It is telling, for example, that research has shown that people are happier if they are at least slightly richer than their friends.

But what if we didn't have friends and colleagues to compare ourselves to? What if our only frame of reference was our personal best? In Neuro Linguistic Programming, broad distinctions are made between predominantly *internally-referenced* people who are generally better at using their own referencing to measure their *success* and those who are more *externally-referenced*, who look for reassurance and confirmation of their abilities from others. Externally-referenced people are more likely to make comparisons with other people as a kind of self-affirmation, but no one lives in a vacuum and everyone has some kind of referencing system to people outside of themselves.

Let me try and put it another way. We all have an actual or imagined *audience* to our lives that gives our actions meaning.

One of the first steps in improving self-esteem is to learn where we currently position ourselves on the line of continuum between being internally-referenced and externally-referenced. Nobody is entirely one type or the other – different patterns will play out with different people at different times. In the workplace, for example, the quality and nature of the relationships we have with colleagues will be coloured by the degree to which we are externally-referenced and the number and strength of comparisons we make in relation to job roles, personality types and status.

Our behaviour will be determined by these perceptions and a conversation with a team member might be very different from a conversation with a line manager, for example. The outcome of the interaction cannot be viewed in isolation from our perceptions of who we are, the boundaries of our role, who our colleague is, the boundaries of their role and the value of our role compared to our colleague's role.

In addition, the perceptions we have and comparisons we make will be based on what we see and hear. However, we see and hear only a small range of other people's behaviour and we need to take this into account when we examine our perceptions.

To pull all of this together, we are making assessments based on a small chunk of information that is internally processed through a system coloured by our own perceptions of self, role, status and personality type! It is no wonder that many people find success a difficult concept to grasp and find it easier to use other people's measures of success than find their own!

The most powerful place on the continuum is in the middle – to be a confident, internally-referenced person who is flexible enough to assess the value of external evidence to support you in making decisions.

So, in addition to recognising our referencing systems, to fully understand success we have to look deep into the essence of our beings and see what it is that makes us who we are. Are we referencing the right stuff? What qualities make us feel good about ourselves? What can we offer to the world around us? What is our personal success gauge? What is our own definition of happiness? We can then accept that our definition of success might look completely different from someone elses, which creates empathy, which is a key facet of emotional intelligence.

The more clarity we have around our definition, the more we have demonstrated personal honesty and the creative imagination to think outside of other people's referencing systems. This also helps us to take responsibility for our own perceptions and definition of reality.

Don't Should on Yourself

We do not do ourselves any favours by using terms like *should have, would have or could have*; in fact you could quite easily eliminate those phrases from your vocabulary. Retrospective regret is a waste of life because you can't turn the clocks back and you can't change what has happened. So my advice is *don't should on yourself*. Turn the experience around, learn from it and think about what you will do better as a result next time.

SUMO

One of the most debilitating and negative things that you can do is to hold onto things and keep dragging up negative baggage from the past. I have learnt a lot from the simple term SUMO - which, simply put, is to "Shut Up and Move On"! When you have some negative nagging feeling that you cannot do anything about and you are allowing it to run out of control like a rat in a maze in your mind, literally tell yourself to let it go and move forward. You will be amazed at how liberating this simple action can be and at the relief to others around you when you let it go and move on to focus on something more positive and constructive.

Coping with the Blues

It may be that there are times that you wake up feeling not so great. You may call it the blues, a let-down after a fun weekend, or just a bad day. We all have those days when we're not feeling tip-top. Should we try to cheer up and reach for a positive attitude, or just go along with feeling a bit flat? This is very different to depression, which we tackle later in the book.

Research indicates there are definite advantages to taking some steps to cheer yourself up. People who feel positive most of the time appear not only to be happier, but are much healthier too.

There are times when cheering up isn't an option. When a tragedy or serious set-back strikes, feeling better personally is the last thing on our minds. In those situations, we're better off allowing the sadness or grief to run its course.

However, for those times when our blues just seem to have settled around our shoulders, for no apparent reason, there are many ways in which we can consciously improve our mental state.

The first and most important thing is to be aware that *you* are the first person that you speak to when you wake up. Your little internal voice will wake you up and tell you how you feel. My advice here is to listen to it and challenge it. This is also the most powerful time of the day and it is really important to refuse the snooze! Another five minutes under the duvet will not help; actually it will probably just make it worse, giving you more time to fester. My advice is to get up and get doing. I am well aware of how challenging that can be; however it is the absolute key to beating the blues.

First thing in the morning is the time to create the foundation or your day – focussing on the positives is great brain gym. In *The Secret,* a book by Rhonda Byrne, there is a great suggestion about adopting an attitude of gratitude. The suggestion is to take a small stone, as a symbol to help you focus, and offer thanks and gratitude for all the things that are good in your life. This helps to get the mind stimulated in a positive way and will influence the rest of your day. Try it – it works really well and is a great habit to adopt.

Another great approach to feeling good is to focus on the day – a great deal of feeling low is because we spend time reflecting on the past and worrying about what we can't do anything about or trying to foretell the future and getting uncomfortable on uncharted territory.

This beautiful Sanskrit proverb is a celebration of each day and the importance of focussing on the here and now:

Look to this day,
The very life of life,
In its brief course lies all
The realities and varieties of existence,
The bliss of growth,
The splendour of action,
The glory of power.
For yesterday is but a dream,
And tomorrow is only a vision.
But today well lived,
Makes every yesterday
A dream of happiness
And every tomorrow
A vision of hope.
Look well, therefore,
To this day.

How to Beat the Blues

✓ Focusing on your breathing keeps your attention on the present moment.
✓ Breathe deeply and slowly, noticing each breath you inhale and exhale.
✓ Laughter is the best medicine. Immerse yourself in humour.
✓ Keep an image of something that makes you happy and look at it when you feel low.
✓ Develop an attitude of gratitude.
✓ A brisk walk or any other form of physical exercise will improve your mood.
✓ Recall a great holiday or a wonderful family reunion.

✓ Reflect on a card or letter someone sent you that was touching and showed they cared for you.
✓ Use one or more of your strengths in some activity to build your self-esteem.
✓ Use positive affirmations.

Visualisation

Visualisation involves allowing your thoughts to extend into an internal video. Playing out a situation in your mind can raise your creativity, change your emotional state and help you focus and reduce tension. It is a very powerful technique and many top performers use visualisation to help focus on successful goal achievement. It's like a mental rehearsal of what you want to happen. Imagining your goals and dreams can lead to you actually experiencing them, because what your mind focuses on, your body will respond by acting upon.

When you visualise, your muscles experience electrical impulses that correspond to the physical event you are imagining. An example is the story of a talented pianist called Liu Chi Kung who was imprisoned for seven years during the Cultural Revolution; when he was released, he played better than ever. When he was interviewed, he was asked how that was possible without him practising. He responded by saying "I did practise, every day. I rehearsed every piece I ever played, note by note, in my mind."

Many coaches now use visualisation as a form of training for competitive games like football and rugby.

Visualisation is not only used by athletes and surgeons, but also in the physical rehabilitation of cancer patients.

Visualisation takes you into a whole new realm – which can be scary and weird, but much safer in the confines of your mind. You can practice examining your success from a new perspective with all sorts of different scenarios! This sets you up for the real thing and, when it actually happens, you'll be ready. Visualisation also allows you to see the big picture, from the perspective of your family, friends and work colleagues.

If you're facing an obstacle you don't understand or haven't ever experienced, your intuition can work its magic. Your mind will reach back into your past for ideas, resources – your intuition will bring forth inspirations that you hadn't previously considered. It will prompt you to turn left or right, or take a whole new road altogether. It will let you know if you're on the right track, and will supply you with motivation and insight.

Motivating Yourself at Work

A few years ago I found myself in a less-than-desirable work situation, doing a job I had no passion for and not really feeling much of a sense of pride and purpose. Clearly my relationship with positivity was somewhat challenged. When I drove to work I used to sit at the traffic lights and will them to go from amber to red so that I would have a few more moments before I had to go into work. It was not a great position to be in and made me really examine what was important in order to manifest the best attitude to work.

The essence of a happy job is to work with what is important to you, the things in life that really attract you, then chart and celebrate your successes and identify how you do well by encouraging feedback on how to do even better. The positive thinker who is unhappy at work takes action to improve things. If you feel negative about your job, try to be more involved, rather than less. The more actively you contribute, the more control you will have.

Creating good working relationships is so important; speaking well about others and congratulating their successes, even when you lose out. Taking responsibility for errors, rather than shifting the blame. Being the work radiator not the work drain. Being a positive force, celebrating when things go well and offering support when things don't go so well. Coming to work with a smile and keep smiling even when you are under pressure. Being enthusiastic rather than negative and critical about your employers or your work. A good way to realistically assess your happiness at work is to ask yourself the following key questions.

- Do I know what is expected of me at work?
- Do I have the materials and equipment I need to do my work right?
- In the last seven days, have I received recognition or praise for good work?

- Does my immediate manager, or someone at work, care about me as a person?
- Is there someone at work who encourages my development?
- At work, do my opinions seem to count?
- Do I truly support the mission/purpose of my company?
- Are my co-workers committed to doing quality work?
- Do I have opportunities at work to learn and grow?

If you have answered no to any of these questions it is important that you take responsibility and challenge why?

Ask yourself whether you are doing your very best. Challenge your views. Ask for feedback and have the courage to give feedback to your manager. A shut up and put up attitude won't make things any better and you will just end up remaining unhappy and affecting others.

The Four P Principle

My own experience highlights to me that there are four key factors that truly affect happiness and productivity at work:

- **Pride:** Pride is about self-dignity. Pride prevents you from doing just enough to get by. Give your work your very best shot and nothing less.
- **Passion:** Just a simple plain "interest" in any work you choose isn't enough. An enthusiasm and

passion for all things worth doing is the key to being motivated and happy.
- **Purpose:** In order to generate that passion, it is important to believe in what you do and have clear goals.
- **Positivity:** Approaching everything you do with a positive attitude and seeing challenges as opportunities.

Achieving Balance

Interestingly enough, when I first started to explore the concept of *Workplace Wellness* and the key enablers, the original working title was *Balance*. Personally, as one who is prone to extremes, the pursuit of balance and bringing some kind of equilibrium into my life has been an interesting voyage of discovery. Like nutrition. We need variety in our diets to keep us healthy and fit. In the same way, we need variety in our lives to keep us mentally and emotionally balanced.

Finding balance is sometimes very elusive, as we struggle to meet the pressures and challenges that are ever-present in modern society. However, there are key physiological, psychological and indeed spiritual requirements that are necessary in order for us to be fulfilled.

In his theory of human needs and fulfilment, Abraham Maslow, the father of humanistic psychology, outlines the basics as food, water, shelter, safety, stability and security. There is also a sense of belonging, of affiliation, of love, followed by self-esteem that stems from achievements, respect and recognition.

Ultimately, we have what Maslow called 'Self-actualisation' - the stage in which you are fulfilled. Maslow himself did not believe that this was about material achievement and emphasis was more on the importance of inner experience of value and meaning.

It would be interesting now for you to take time to consider how you define personal success and how this differs from the kind of achievement that you feel is expected of you. Self-definement is key in order for us to feel a sense of robust self-esteem and the courage to explore our own potential.

> *Attitude is a little thing that makes a big difference*
>
> *—Winston Churchill*

How to Work Wonders with Your Attitude

✓ Take personal responsibility for everything you think, feel and do.

✓ Refuse the Snooze on work days – get up and get going.

✓ Make sure that your internal voice is having a positive chat with you.

✓ Look in the mirror and tell yourself that you are feeling good.

✓ Be positive when you respond to other people.

✓ Try not to infect others with your NAGs.

✓ Try not to should on yourself!

✓ Balance your internal and external referencing.

✓ Avoid comparing yourself to others.

✓ Be a radiator, not a drain.

✓ Slay the Doom goblin.

✓ Feed your dinner table of emotions positive thoughts.

✓ Turn problems into opportunities.

✓ Get rid of your NITs!

✓ Make sure that you have balance in your life.

✓ Use SUMO – shut up and move on.

✓ Live each day how you would like to repeat it.

CHAPTER TWO
EXERCISE & NUTRITION

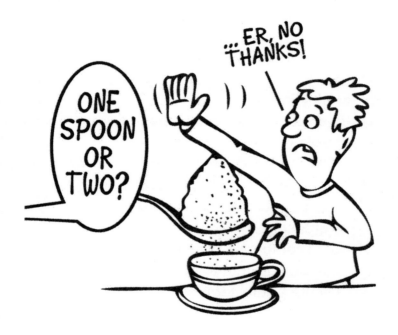

The greatest wealth is health

Virgil

I mentioned in the previous chapter that your brain is your most valuable asset. So, given the choice, would you want yours to be carried around in a bin liner or a Rolls Royce?

I am working on the assumption that you would choose the Rolls Royce! So, providing that was your answer let me ask you something else. If you were in possession of such a fine vehicle would you take it rally driving? Hopefully not. However, if your body is the Rolls Royce that chauffeurs around your most valuable asset, can you honestly say that you drive it, fuel it and service it in the best possible way?

In the UK alone we consume over one billion pounds worth of ready–made meals per year and spend three billion pounds on fast foods. Ironically enough, we then spend over two million pounds on diet products!

Six out of ten people are now considered to be obese with an increasing amount of illness linked to poor nutrition and bad eating habits. Our life style is becoming more and more sedentary with people taking less than the recommended amount of exercise of thirty minutes a day.

Please don't think for one minute that I am going to take the moral high ground here. I have certainly been there myself and have on occasions treated my body more like an amusement arcade than a temple. I have learnt, however, through experience and raised awareness that a healthy body equals a healthy mind and, personally, I have found that the health benefits, increased energy and general feel-good factor have made a significant difference. Mental and physical health work hand in hand and one does not effectively work without the support of the other.

Health in the 21st Century

According to the World Health Organisation, cardiovascular diseases are the leading cause of death in the world. These are diseases of the heart and blood vessels that can cause heart attacks and stroke. That is the bad news. The good news is that, in most cases, it is preventable. Apart from a few genetically-inherited cases, there is nothing natural about dying from a heart attack.

Many cultures do not experience a high incidence of heart attacks. For example, by middle age, British people have nine times as much heart disease as the Japanese, although the Japanese are now showing signs of catching up. Autopsies performed on the mummified remains of Egyptians who died about 3000 BC showed deposits in the arteries but no actual blockages that would result in a stroke or heart attack. In the 1930s, heart attacks were so rare it took a specialist to make the diagnosis.

Even more worrying is the fact that heart disease is occurring at a younger and younger age. Clearly something about our lifestyle, diet or even environment has changed radically in the last sixty years to bring on this modern epidemic.

After cardiovascular disease and cancer, diabetes is the third largest killer and this is directly attributable to obesity, diet and lifestyle. Our current eating patterns are not making us any healthier.

There is no getting away from the fact that if you are overweight, you will feel tired, lethargic, suffer from digestive problems and have aching joints because your body has to take the strain of the extra load. A pill may take away the pain, however it does not get rid of the problem.

Your Amazing Machine

The concept of your body as a machine is the product of the thinking of philosophers such as Newton and Descartes and of the Industrial Revolution, which envisioned a clockwork universe and man as a thinking machine. The way in which we fuel our machine, however, has deteriorated quite significantly.

Until a couple of hundred years ago, our ancestors had spent millions of years being hunter-gatherers and tens of thousands of years being peasant farmers, only to be propelled into the new towns and cities to fuel the need for labour during the Industrial Revolution. The diet the new industrial workers were fed consisted of fat, sugar and refined flour. A biscuit or a cake is a good example.

Flour was refined so that it would not go off and cheap energy-providing food was considered fuel in the same way that a car needs petrol. Not surprisingly, health declined. By about 1900, people had started to be smaller than in earlier generations. This led to the discovery of protein – the factor in food needed for growth. Sugar for energy, and protein for muscle. With this concept, the Western diet of high sugar, fat and protein was born.

Your body is an amazing machine, your heart beats, your blood goes around, your lungs breathe and your digestive system merrily gurgles away. Most of the time, especially when we are younger, we don't even need to think about all those bodily functions and we take them for granted. However, as we grow older, we become increasingly aware of how important it is to look after our bodies, especially as we are now living longer and physical preservation is a key consideration.

Another area of illness is depression. About one in ten of us will develop some form of depression in our lives, and one in fifty has severe depression. This has now been recognised as a very real medical condition and this number is increasing. If depression continues, it could be the leading cause of disability and ill health around the world, with nearly a million people already taking their own lives each year. Exercise and nutrition can play a very important part in combating this illness. It is also important to seek help from your GP if you think you may be depressed.

You Are Special

First of all, let's get one thing straight – there is nobody on this planet who is exactly the same as you. There are many principles that apply to us all as members of the human race – for example, we all need to move and fuel ourselves to keep going; however, to what extent will vary from each individual. You are essentially the evolutionary dynamics that you have inherited from your parents and the genetically-inherited strengths and weaknesses. The complex interaction of these factors ensures that each individual is born unique although clearly similar to other people.

Understanding ourselves and what works best for us is the first step to better health and personal performance. There are however some key aspects of exercise and nutrition that are fundamental to all of us and this chapter is about helping you to raise awareness of the benefits of what we can do to improve our health.

Exercise

Before we delve into the subject of nutrition and diet, let's examine the concept of exercise. There really is no way around it: the lack of physical activity is probably the greatest reason why obesity figures are rising. You need to increase your physical activity if you want to lose weight; however, exercise is also good for your all-round health and wellbeing. As the biggest proportion of the population have non-physical jobs, it is easy to become disassociated from your body. Getting back in touch with it through exercise will increase your self esteem and feelings of control, as well as your energy levels, metabolism and overall fitness.

I saw a strap line the other day that said: *"Energy – the more you give the more you get"* which I thought sums up exercise very well. People who exercise regularly are likely to live longer and enjoy a better quality of life. In fact, studies have shown that being physically unfit is just as dangerous as smoking in terms of lowering life expectancy.

Regular exercise also improves mental and emotional health. The chemicals and hormones that are released in the brain through exercise can help deal with stress and promote happiness.

The Benefits of Exercise

- Reduces the risk of premature death.
- Reduces the risk of developing heart disease.
- Reduces high blood pressure or the risk of developing high blood pressure.
- Reduces high cholesterol or the risk of developing high cholesterol.
- Reduces the risk of developing colon cancer and breast cancer.
- Reduces the risk of developing diabetes.

- Reduces or maintains body weight or body fat.
- Builds and maintains healthy muscles, bones, and joints.
- Reduces depression and anxiety.
- Improves psychological wellbeing.
- Enhances work, recreation, and sport performance.

Sometimes, the very mention of the word exercise makes most people want to reach for the chocolate. There is something about the word that can conjure up gyms, breathless running or crowded aerobics classes that puts many people off.

The good news is that you don't even have to go to a gym for hours and hours at a time. In reality, as little as half an hour of moderate activity every day, such as brisk walking, can be enough to improve health and fitness. There are many different ways to exercise and it is possible to find something to suit any kind of lifestyle.

Simply put, you need to get off your bum and start moving. Be really honest with yourself now – at work do you walk up the stairs or take the lift? How many car journeys do you take door to door when really you could walk at least part of the way? Do you send an email when you could walk across the office to deliver the message in person? If you really *sit* and think about it, how active are you?

Almost every function in our bodies depends partly on exercise for its optimum function – our digestion and elimination, our lungs and breathing, our heart and cardiovascular system and not least of all our weight management.

Remember too that exercise helps you to make a very positive investment for your future. While we worry about our pensions and make provision materially do we also consider whether we are going to be healthy and active enough in later life to enjoy our retirement. We are living longer these days - therefore our long term health is an increasingly concerning issues. My Dad is an inspiration and shining example of the benefits of exercise. Having battled cancer and managed bouts of depression throughout his lifetime, he is an absolute advocate of - *a healthy body equals a healthy mind*.

At seventy six, he goes to the gym every weekday and races a single-handed boat at weekends and is full of beans and vitality!

Get Walking

It's free and even better when using nature's gym – the great outdoors. Walking is essential for your health. It exercises virtually all your muscle groups, with all the major muscles being used at the same time, providing you aim to walk at a brisk pace and swing your arms to help propel you along.

Walking increases your heart-rate and ensures that your blood is being pumped around your body at a faster pace than when you are sitting still. The heart itself is a muscle and needs imposed exercise.

Government guidelines recommend that you should aim to walk 10,000 steps a day. It may sound a lot but 50 years ago this would have been the norm for every one of us. Today most overweight people are often walking less than 3000 steps per day and it is now estimated that we eat over twice as much as we did 50 years ago.

Walking is also the perfect antidote to depression and anxiety. It can aid the release of serotonin, a brain chemical that helps to rejuvenate your mood. This is why so many people experience a natural high and lift in mood after exercising. It would be great if doctors could prescribe thirty minutes of brisk walking a day; this would be a very beneficial and positive self medication.

Walking deserves special focus because it is often the easiest, most convenient and best exercise for many people.

- No special equipment is required except a good pair of walking shoes.
- It costs nothing.
- It is non-competitive, so feelings of not being as good as others don't arise.
- You can walk anytime and anywhere that is safe.
- Walking in the countryside or in parks that have natural settings has the added benefit of communion with nature.
- You can walk in whatever you happen to be wearing. You don't have to change your clothes or shower after walking.

- It is very unlikely that you will incur the type of overuse injuries that occur with some other types of exercise.

Recently I have discovered the wonders of a pedometer - a small device that you can clip onto your waist band to measure the amount of steps you achieve each day. It is a great incentive and, by setting yourself a goal, you can measure and keep track of your steps.

Wearing your pedometer to work will act as an additional incentive to keep you moving about. You can set yourself a specific number of steps that you would like to achieve at work. Encouraging your colleagues to wear one too will promote energy levels.

The pedometer makes expediency and functionality come together for a more accurate walking exercise. It works through a sensor run by software attached to the apparatus. As you take a step forward and walk, the pedometer calculates your tread and every stride to provide you with a fairly accurate figure. Since people are of different stature, pedometers offer a precise measurement regardless of a person's height. You can use whatever types of pedometer you like; these are all dependent on your preference and the kind of lifestyle you lead. If you are an office worker wanting to get out of the typical deskbound activity, you can walk around and perform some exercise without anyone noticing by means of purchasing a premium pedometer. For those who prefer aerobics and jogging, a pedometer that measures both jogging strides and aerobic moves is better.

You may not have a have an outrageously excessive diet; however, if you are not moving, you will put on weight. It's a very simple mathematical equation - calories in versus calories out. You can try all the latest diet crazes in the world but in the end your success and failure will boil down to how you balance this simple equation.

Choosing the Right Exercise Programme for You

When setting up an exercise programme that is right for you, focus on what you enjoy. Whether it is swimming, dancing, working out on exercise machines or team sports ...any kind of exercise that you enjoy is acceptable! You can do the same kind of exercise every day or vary it according to the weather. It may help if you make a list of exercise options and post it in a convenient place. Then you can look at the list and decide each day how you are going to get your exercise. This makes exercise more interesting for some of us.

Like most people, you may have had difficulty beginning or sticking to an exercise programme. Perhaps one or several of the following suggestions would help.

How to Stick to an Exercise Programme

✓ Consider your exercise time as fun or "play" time, not as work.

✓ Ask friends and/or family members to exercise with you.
✓ Reward yourself each time you exercise.
✓ Schedule exercise at the same time each day to provide structure and routine.
✓ Avoid sabotaging yourself. If you miss a day, don't give up and stop exercising.
✓ Keep an exercise log describing what you did and how you felt.

Exercising at Work

It may be hard to find time to exercise, especially for those of us who work in an office. Exercising at work may seem impossible, but it's one option for staying fit and keeping your energy up. It takes some creativity, but there are opportunities to exercise at work if you pay attention. All it takes is a little planning and some inspiration to squeeze in a little movement throughout the day.

How to Exercise at Work

✓ Take the stairs, when you can, instead of the lift.
✓ If you drive to work, park some distance from the entrance door.
✓ Cycle to work in good weather if you live close enough.
✓ Walk around the office when you can.
✓ Sit on an exercise ball instead of a chair.
✓ Set an alarm to go off every hour to remind you to stand up and move.
✓ Use a pedometer and keep track of how many steps you take.

- Deliver documents or messages to co-workers in person rather than by email.
- Get a headset for your phone so you can move around while you talk.

Be creative. Any movement is better than none. Adding short bouts of exercise throughout the day will help you burn more calories and will also reduce stress.

Your boss may also not have considered how much more productive his or her employees would be with a little exercise. Why not suggest the following:

How to Make Your Work-Environment Exercise-Friendly

✓ Work with local gyms to provide membership discounts for employees.
✓ Work with local personal trainers to provide monthly seminars.
✓ Introduce walking meetings.
✓ Set up daily or weekly walks during lunch or after work.
✓ Encourage sponsoring a charity and set up a company walkathon.
✓ Staff to wear pedometers at work.
✓ Be active. If the boss exercises, employees will take their own health more seriously.

Even if your immediate manager isn't interested in exercise, you can do a lot to get others involved in working out.

The Work Workout

This basic work workout offers stretches for your arms, wrists and back (the body parts that suffer most from sitting and typing all day). You'll also find some basic strength training exercises you can do while sitting at your desk or standing. Use whatever time you can find and do the exercises throughout the day.

N.B. Precautions - See your doctor before trying this workout if you have any injuries, illnesses or conditions. Make sure the chair you use is stable. If you have wheels, push it against a wall to make sure it won't roll away.

Equipment Needed - A chair and a water bottle or light-medium dumbbell.

How to Work Out in the Workplace

✓ **Wrist Stretch**
Extend arm in front, palm up and grab the fingers with other hand. Gently pull the fingers towards you to stretch the forearm, holding for 20-30 seconds. Repeat on the other side.

✓ **Wrist & Forearm**
Press hands together in front of chest, elbows bent and parallel to the floor. Gently bend wrists to the right and left for 10 repetitions.

✓ **Lower Back Stretch**
Sit tall and place the left arm behind left hip. Gently twist to the left, using the right hand to deepen the

stretch, holding for 20-30 seconds. Repeat on the other side.

✓ Hip Flexion

Sit tall with the abs in and lift the left foot off the floor a few inches, knee bent. Hold for 2 seconds, lower and repeat for 16 repetitions. Repeat on the other side.

✓ Leg Extension

Sit tall with the abs in and extend the left leg until it is level with hip, squeezing the quadriceps. Hold for 2 seconds, lower and repeat for 16 reps. Repeat on the other side.

✓ Chair Squat

While sitting, lift up until your hips are just hovering over the chair, arms out for balance. Hold for 2-3 seconds, stand all the way up and repeat for 16 repetitions.

✓ Dips

Make sure chair is stable and place hands next to hips. Move hips in front of chair and bend the elbows, lowering the body until the elbows are at 90 degrees. Push back up and repeat for 16 repetitions.

✓ One-Leg Squat

Make sure the chair is stable and take one foot slightly in front of the other. Use the hands for leverage as you push up into a one-legged squat, hovering just over the chair and keeping the other leg on the floor for balance. Lower and repeat; only coming a few inches off the chair for 12 repetitions. Repeat on the other side.

✓ Front Raise to Triceps Press

Sit tall with the abs in and hold a full water bottle in the left hand. Lift the bottle up to shoulder level, pause, and then continue lifting all the way up over the head. When the arm is next to the ear, bend the elbow, taking the water bottle behind you and contracting the triceps. Straighten the arm and lower down, repeating 12 times on each arm.

✓ Bicep Curl

Hold water bottle in right hand and, with abs in and spine straight, curl bottle towards shoulder for 16 repetitions. Repeat other side.

✓ Side Bends

Hold a water bottle with both hands and stretch it up over the head, arms straight. Gently bend towards the left as far as you can, contracting the abs. Come back to centre and repeat to the right. Complete 10 repetitions (bending to the right and left is one rep).

✓ Abdominal Twists

Hold the water bottle at chest level and, keeping the knees and hips forward, gently twist to the left as far as you comfortably can, feeling the abs contract. Twist back to centre and move to the left for a total of 10 repetitions. Don't force it or you may end up with a back injury.

In Summary

Stretching at your desk and standing up when you answer the phone is also positive practice. Any kind of exercise and movement that you can do through the day will be very helpful in keeping you active and energised.

Nutrition - You Are What You Eat

No matter who you are or where you live, the very fact that you are alive depends on you eating and keeping hydrated. Even the sight and smell of food can trigger the release of a pleasurable and rewarding chemical called dopamine in your brain.

However, while a delicious meal and a drink can be one of the most satisfying sensory experiences, it is also responsible for some of our greatest health problems.

You are essentially what you eat. Each human being is made up of roughly 63 per cent water, 22 per cent protein, 13 per cent fat and 2 per cent minerals and vitamins. Every single molecule comes from the food you eat and the water you drink. Eating the highest quality food in the right quantities helps you to achieve your highest potential for health, vitality and freedom from disease.

However, many people who believe that they have a healthy well balanced diet with all the necessary nutrients are misguided. Part of the problem is propaganda and consumerism. It is not easy in today's society (in which food production is inextricably linked to profit). Refining foods makes them last longer, which makes them more profitable yet, at the same time, deficient in essential nutrients.

The food industry has gradually conditioned us to eat sweet foods. Sugar sells and it has been suggested that sugar is more addictive than heroin. As our lives speed up, we spend less time preparing fresh food and become even more reliant on readymade meals from companies more concerned about *their* own profit than *our* health.

In Patrick Holford's book *The Optimum Nutrition Bible* (one of the best books that I have read and would strongly recommend) the importance of nutrition and its impact on our health is stated as being paramount to our overall wellbeing.

The *optimum nutrition* approach is not new. In AD 390 Hippocrates said "Let food be thy medicine and medicine be thy food". In the early 20th century Thomas Edison said "The doctor of the future will no longer treat the human frame with drugs but rather will cure and prevent disease with nutrition".

What is a Well Balanced Diet?

Nothing in Western society really teaches us to be healthy. Apart from any wisdom that our parents may impart, we are not really taught how to be healthy. The media has embarked upon many well intentioned health campaigns; however, so many mixed messages are now sent out about what is good for you, and what is not, that many of us are left in a state of confusion about what constitutes a healthy, well-balanced diet.

Having worked with some nutritional experts who have conducted corporate fitness programmes, it is quite concerning how poor some individuals' knowledge of nutrition is. For example, when analysing one senior executive's diet due to high blood sugar levels, she had been under the impression that her vitamin intake was good because she drank a bottle of Ribena a day, however did not eat any fruit or vegetables!

How many times have you followed a diet without really understanding the difference between a protein and a complex carbohydrate, what each of them do in the body or in which foods they are found? No dietary plan is ever going to be truly successful if you don't have a little background knowledge. So here is a basic low-down on which nutrients are found in what.

Proteins

The word *protein* comes from the Greek word *protos* meaning *first things.* Three quarters of all the solid matter in your body is protein, which forms the building blocks of our bodies. Without sufficient proteins, the body actually breaks down faster than it repairs itself.

While a lack of protein in our diet depresses all our functions, a long term high protein diet places a strain on the body as it causes high levels of acidity. This can be harmful to the body's tissues. Catabolism is the breaking down of body tissue; the body has several buffering systems against this and will use calcium as a main buffering mineral. The calcium has to be taken out of bones and teeth. Consequently one of the long term effects of a high protein diet is a higher risk of osteoporosis. This illustrates how important it is to maintain a well balanced diet.

Carbohydrates

There are two main types of carbohydrates: complex and simple. Basically, complex carbohydrates are those in whole grain, and simple carbohydrates are those that have been processed and broken down. Examples of complex carbohydrates are brown rice, wholegrain bread, porridge oats and muesli, while simple carbohydrates include commercial cereals, white bread, bagels, cakes, pastries and biscuits. Most simple carbohydrates also have added sugars and often include preservatives because they are more likely to become stale.

The role of carbohydrates is to produce energy. All carbohydrates are broken down into glucose molecules and are the body's preferred source of fuel.

Fats

The body needs a certain amount of fats for various vital functions. The brain and the nervous system are made up of around 60 per cent fats. All your hormones are created out of essential fats and the skin is lubricated and protected by them. Your skin is your largest bodily organ and is your first line of defence so a lack of fats in your diet will actually show in dry scaly skin. Your skin is a great tell tale sign of whether or not you are eating the *right* kind of fats.

Polyunsaturated fats and mono-unsaturated fats are very beneficial to the brain and nervous system and include olive oil, pumpkin seed oil, walnut oil, nuts and seeds and tahini (sesame seed spread). Also the Omega-3 and Omega-6 essential fatty acids that are talked about so much these days are vital for the cognitive function. They are also responsible for some of the anti-inflammatory processes in the body. They are found primarily in oily fish, as well as most nuts and seeds.

Fibre

Rural Africans eat about 55 grams of dietary fibre a day compared to the UK average intake of 22 grams of fibre and have the lowest incidence of bowel diseases. The ideal intake is not less than 35 grams a day. It is relatively easy to take in this amount of fibre – which absorbs water into the digestive tract making the food contents bulkier and easier to pass through the body – by eating whole grains, vegetables, fruit, nuts and seeds on a daily basis. Cereal fibre and linseed is especially good for avoiding constipation.

Vitamins

Although required in smaller amounts than fat, protein or carbohydrates, vitamins are extremely important to our diets. They stimulate *enzymes* which in turn make all the body processes happen. Vitamins are needed to balance hormones, produce energy, boost the immune system, make healthy skin and protect our arteries. They are also vital for our brain, nervous system and just about every body process.

Minerals

Like vitamins, minerals are essential. Calcium, magnesium and phosphorus help make up the bones and teeth. Nerve signals, which are vital for the brain and muscles, depend on calcium, magnesium, sodium and potassium. Other minerals include chromium for controlling blood sugar levels and selenium and zinc which are essential for bodily repair and the immune system. Mineral rich foods include: kale, cabbage, root vegetables, fresh fruit and vegetables and whole foods such as lentils, beans and whole grains.

Given below are the names of the various vitamins and minerals that are required by the human body and some examples of foods that are rich in these.

Vitamin B6

Vitamin B6 helps in metabolising protein and amino acids and in converting other amino acids into hormones; builds red blood cells and antibodies and maintains the central nervous system. This can be found in avocados, bananas, chicken, cabbage, green and red peppers, lentils, salmon, soybeans, steak, sweet potatoes, trout, wheat germ, yellow fin tuna, cauliflower and chickpeas.

Vitamin B12

Vitamin B12 is needed to produce red blood cells. It helps build and maintain myelin, a protective sheath found around nerves and synthesizes your DNA. It can be found in clams, crab, herring, liver, mackerel, mussels, oysters, salmon, trout, eggs, steak and yogurt.

Vitamin C

Vitamin C helps build and maintain collagen, which aids wound healing. It is also good for healthy blood vessels, scavenging free radicals, metabolising certain amino acids, stimulating the adrenal function, metabolising cholesterol and boosting the immune system. It can be found in broccoli, Brussel sprouts, cantaloupe, green and red peppers, guava, kale, kiwi, lemons, oranges, papaya, strawberries, blackberries, peas and tomatoes.

Calcium

Calcium builds strong bones and teeth. It plays a role in the transmission of nerve impulses, in blood clotting and in smooth muscle contraction and also helps to regulate heart rhythm. It can be found in cheese, cabbage, beans, ricotta, sesame seeds, soybeans, tofu, yogurt, artichokes and trout.

Carbohydrates

Carbohydrates are the body's main source of energy as previously mentioned and help to regulate the metabolism of proteins and fats. Positive carbohydrates can be found in apples, black beans, chickpeas, kidney beans, lentils, pinto beans, quinoa, sweet potatoes, blackberries, butternut squash, corn, parsnips, peas, raspberries and wheat germ.

Copper

Copper is needed to manufacture red blood cells and collagen also aids in the absorption and transport of iron. It can be found in liver, wild oysters, crab, lobster, squid, Brazil nuts, cashews, chickpeas, clams, hazelnuts, lentils, beans, quinoa, mushrooms, sesame seeds and soybeans.

Vitamin D

Vitamin D is needed for the absorption of calcium and phosphorus. It can be found in halibut, herring, mackerel, oysters, tuna, mushrooms, eggs and hard cheese.

Vitamin E

Vitamin E prevents damage to cell membranes and keeps bad cholesterol from oxidising, which is the first step in the build-up of blocked arteries. It can be found in wheat germ, sunflower seeds, almonds and almond oil, asparagus, avocados, eel, hazelnuts, mangos, soybeans, blueberries, Brazil nuts, broccoli, lobster, nectarines and papaya.

Fibre

Fibre helps to lower cholesterol and to stabilise blood sugar levels, it provides steady source of energy and gives bulk to stools and speeds the passage of waste through the intestines. It can be found in black beans, chickpeas, kidney beans, lentils, apples, artichokes, avocados, blackberries, carrots, corn, guava, parsnips, peanuts, peas, quinoa, raspberries, sunflower seeds, sweet potatoes and wheat germ.

Folate

Folate metabolises protein and converts many amino acids, it also forms the nucleic acids for DNA and is needed to produce red blood cells. It can be found in chickpeas, kidney beans, lentils, liver, artichokes, asparagus, avocados, beetroot, blackberries, cabbage, green beans, mustard greens, oranges, papaya, sunflower seeds, tofu, wheat germ, seeds, peanuts and salmon.

Iron

Iron is needed to form haemoglobin and to transfer oxygen from the lungs to every cell in the body and used by several enzymes to produce energy. It can be found in soybeans, kidney beans, lentils, liver, mussels, mushrooms, oysters, pine nuts, pumpkin seeds, shrimp, steak, green beans and pistachio nuts.

Vitamin K

Vitamin K is needed for proper blood clotting. It can be found in broccoli, endive, kale, spinach, watercress, avocados and kiwi.

Magnesium

Magnesium aids in muscle relaxation, helps metabolise carbohydrates and proteins and activates more than 300 enzymes. It can be found in almonds, artichokes, avocados, black beans, butternut squash, corn, halibut, mackerel, peas and tofu.

Manganese

Manganese is needed to metabolise glucose, to synthesise cholesterol and fatty acids, to build strong bones, and to make urea (a waste product found in urine). It can be found in mussels, pineapple, blackberries, brown rice, pine nuts, raspberries, soybeans, tofu, walnuts and chestnuts.

Niacin

Niacin is needed to break down carbohydrates, fats, and proteins and helps in the formation of red blood cells and steroids. It also keeps the skin, digestive tract, and nervous system healthy. It can be found in Marmite, avocados, barley, brown and white rice, corn, ground beef, lamb, mushrooms, peas, salmon, tuna and turkey.

Pantothenic Acid

Pantothenic acid supports the adrenal glands and is important to healthy skin and the nervous system. It also helps metabolise carbohydrates and fats into energy and is needed to make fatty acids, cholesterol and steroids. It can be found in avocados, chicken, eggs, lentils, lobster, mushrooms, salmon, sunflower seeds, wheat germ and yoghurt.

Phosphorus

Phosphorus is needed to build bones and teeth, it is also essential to the metabolism of carbohydrates and fats and to the synthesising of proteins. It can be found in almonds, artichokes, corn, eggs, peas, and pumpkin seeds, salmon, sesame seeds, sweet, swordfish, tofu, trout, tuna, turkey and yogurt.

Potassium

Potassium works with sodium to maintain the body's fluid balance. It also helps to metabolise carbohydrates and synthesise protein, and to transmit nerve impulses. It can be found in bananas, butternut squash, cantaloupe, cabbage, cod, halibut, herring, honeydew melon, papaya, pinto beans, quinoa, soybeans and tomatoes.

Protein

Protein is needed to form, maintain and repair cells. It is used as building blocks for hormones, enzymes and antibodies. It can be found in beans, lentils, lobster, oyster mushrooms, cheese, peanuts, peas, pine nuts, pork, pumpkin seeds, ricotta, salmon, steak, swordfish, tofu, trout, tuna, turkey, walnuts and eggs.

Riboflavin

Riboflavin helps metabolise carbohydrates and fats into energy it is needed for healthy hair, skin, nails, vision, and cell growth. It can be found in marmite, almonds, avocados, clams, eggs, cheese, ham, herring, mackerel, mushrooms, peas, pork, squid, sweet potatoes, wheat germ, wild salmon, bananas, cheese, lentils, mangos, raspberries and cheese.

Selenium

Selenium protects cell membranes from free radicals and helps eliminate certain heavy metals. It can be found in couscous, liver, mackerel, shrimp, swordfish, tuna, wheat germ, brown rice, eggs, beef, mushrooms, pork and soya beans.

Thiamine

Thiamine is needed to metabolise glucose into energy and to convert carbohydrates into fat, it is important for a healthy heart and nervous system. It can be found in asparagus, avocados, black beans, Brazil nuts, brown and white rice, corn, lentils, grapes and pineapple.

Zinc

Zinc helps the liver detoxify alcohol. It also bolsters the immune system and is important for energy production. It helps maintain healthy skin cells aids, protein digestion, and regulates normal insulin activity. It can be found in crab, black beans, chicken, chickpeas, lamb, lentils, lobster, mussels, peanuts, wild rice, yogurt and nuts.

Water - The Elixir of Life

I have just recently discovered a book called *Your Body's Many Cries for Water* written by Dr. F. Batmanghelidj. Dr Batman (or Dr B as he has affectionately been called) has produced some pioneering work that shows that *Unintentional Chronic Dehydration* (UCD) can contribute to and even produce pain and many degenerative diseases that can be prevented and treated by increasing water intake on a regular basis.

Under the grim conditions of captivity in Evin prison in Tehran, Dr Batman found what he believed to be a new and remarkable treatment for the pain of peptic ulcers.

The treatment was simply several glasses of water taken at prescribed regular intervals. Dr Batman discovered the treatment largely by accident and was able to examine about 3,000 patients and follow the medical fate of more than 600, mostly fellow prisoners.

"I was lucky to have been able to make my observations ... when I was waiting clarification of my own situation," Dr Batman said in a guest editorial in the Journal of Clinical Gastroenterology.

It started with one of his patients suffering unbearable ulcer pain late at night. The doctor treated him with a pint of water, evidently because nothing else was available at that hour.

"His pain became less severe and then disappeared completely after eight minutes," said Dr Batman. He was so impressed that he prescribed two glasses of water, six times a day, and achieved a clinical cure of the ulcer attack during the patient's stay of a few months in the prison. After that, Dr Batman used the treatment with other prisoners, reducing the amount to one glass half an hour before eating and another glass two and a half hours later.

Gradually, the treatment came into use throughout the prison as its effectiveness became clear in patients whose chronic ulcers were exacerbated by the stress of prison life.

Two thirds of our bodies consist of water, which is therefore our most important nutrient. Water is the basis of all life and that includes your body. Your muscles that move your body are 75% water, your blood that transport nutrients is 82% water, your lungs that provide your oxygen are 90% water, your brain that is the control centre of your body is 76% water and even your bones are 25% water.

The body loses about 1.5 litres of water a day through the skin, lungs and via our kidneys through urine, ensuring that our toxic substances are eliminated from the body. We also eliminate a third of a litre of water a day when glucose is burnt for energy. The ideal intake therefore is around 1.5 litres of water a day and more if you do more exercise. This is on top of water you may get through alkaline foods e.g. fruits and veg with high water content.

According to Dr Batman, most of us are in a state of dehydration most of the time and some of the biggest telltale signs of lack of hydration is low energy, headaches and irritability. Water can have a great effect on our energy at work and a suggestion is to keep a large bottle of water with you and try to set yourself a goal of drinking it all by the end of the day. Try it, it really does work wonders.

Eating a balanced diet with the right amount of nutrients and minerals is essential for the long term investment in your health. There is an assortment of fad diets on the market and, in the UK alone; we spend over 2 million pounds on diet products each year. Six in ten people in Britain are either overweight or obese with the statistics rising as we read.

While we are surrounded with tempting media-hyped products packed full of sugar and other addictive flavourings, it is a challenge not to be tempted into over indulgence. As I already mentioned, if we work on the 80/20 rule and stick to healthy eating 80% of the time we will make some great progress in improving our diets.

How to Eat a Balanced Diet Every Day

✓ Try to eat one heaped tablespoon of ground seeds or one tablespoon of cold pressed seed oil.
✓ Eat at least two servings of beans, lentils, tofu (soya) or seed vegetables.
✓ Eat three to five pieces of fresh fruit such as apples, pears, bananas, berries, melon or citrus fruit.
✓ Eat four servings of whole grains such as brown rice, millet, rye, oats, whole wheat, corn, quinoa as cereal, breads and pasta.
✓ Eat five root vegetables such as watercress, carrots, sweet potato, broccoli, spinach, green beans, peas and peppers.
✓ Drink eight glasses of water, diluted juices, herb or fruit teas.
✓ Eat whole, organic, raw food as often as you can.
✓ For added energy and support supplement your diet with a high strength multi vitamin especially in winter to build your immunity.

What to Avoid

There are certain foods and drinks that we would be best avoiding wherever possible.

Refined Sugar

While a cat likes the taste of proteins, humans are principally attracted to the taste of carbohydrates – sweetness. The inherent attraction toward sweetness worked well for early man because most things in nature that are sweet are not poisonous. Unfortunately, however, we have learnt to extract the sweetness from nature and leave the goodness behind.

White sugar, for example, has 90% of its vitamins and minerals removed. Without sufficient vitamins and minerals, our metabolism becomes inefficient contributing to poor health and weight management issues.

Sugary foods can also compromise your immune system. Research has shown that white blood cells are less efficient at fighting illness when exposed to refined sugar. A diet high in refined sugar will also raise your insulin levels quickly, which can lead to many other health problems. You will also lack energy as a result of these sugar spikes and the drop in blood sugar that follows.

Fruit contains a simpler and more natural sugar called *fructose, which* needs no digesting however needs to be converted into *glucose* first which slows down the metabolism, so you can balance your blood sugar levels more effectively. Keeping your blood sugar levels balanced is probably the most important factor in maintaining balanced even energy levels.

The average American consumes an astounding 2-3 pounds of sugar each week. In the last 20 years, sugar consumption in the U.S. has increased and prior to the turn of this century, the average consumption was only 5 lbs per person per year!

In 2003, the United Nations and the World Health Organization released guidelines that sugar should account for no more than 10% of our daily calories. In a 2,000-calorie-a-day diet, that's just 200 calories or eight heaped teaspoons of table sugar at 25 calories each. A single can of fizzy drink is the equivalent of 10 teaspoons, which would put you well over the recommended amount (and that is not to mention all the hidden refined sugars in processed food).

It's no secret that obesity and weight-related illnesses are on the rise in many countries and this is directly attributed to our diets and lifestyle. Our bodies simply aren't able to cope with such high sugar levels and this is why illnesses like diabetes and heart disease are at an all time high. Cutting the excess sugar out of your diet is one of the best things you can do for your body.

I have recently given up refined sugar all together and the difference to my health, energy and mood has been quite remarkable.

Artificial Sweeteners

When people decide to lose weight, one of the first changes many make to their diet is to add artificial sweeteners in place of sugar. We have been told by the government that artificial sweeteners are safe, but there are a great many indications and current research that suggests the contrary. Aspartame, for example, is made up of three components: fifty percent is phenylalanine, forty percent is aspartic acid and ten percent is methanol or wood alcohol and was discovered as an ulcer drug, not a sweetener.

Side Effects of Artificial Sweeteners

Headaches - These are one of the side effects associated with almost every artificial sweetener on the market. It is also part of the condition known as Aspartame Sickness which refers to a collection of ailments seemingly caused by the consumption of that particular artificial sweetener.

Gastrointestinal Problems - Many of the most popular artificial sweeteners have also been associated with nausea, vomiting and diarrhœa. Usually these problems occur after high levels of the product are consumed or in people who are sensitive to the products. Foods containing sugar alcohols such as sorbitol must be labelled to warn consumers about these problems.

Allergic Reactions - Some consumers have reported allergic reactions to some of the artificial sweeteners available. These reactions have been relatively mild including headaches, skin rashes and similar symptoms.

Panic Attacks - Just as too much sugar can cause nervous agitation, people who consume some types of artificial sweeteners have reported experiencing panic attacks, which include symptoms such as racing heart beats, shortness of breath, feelings of impending doom and more. People who have a tendency to have panic attacks may also have their attacks triggered by an intake of these sweeteners.

Cell Damage - Some of the research on artificial sweeteners has also shown that they can do some damage to cells. For this reason, infants, children and teenagers should have their intake of artificial sweeteners limited.

Central Nervous System Disorders - Research suggests that Aspartame may also be one of the causes or triggers of many serious central nervous system disorders and depression.

Cancer - One of the biggest concerns about these artificial sweeteners has been cancer. There is some research to suggest a higher incidence of bladder cancer (saccharin), cancer of the reproductive organs (aspartame) and more. Research on these connections is continuing.

The best thing to do is avoid all artificial and chemical sweetener substitutes. They have NO food value, trick the body into thinking it is eating something sweet and they have toxic by-products which can produce harmful side effects.

Caffeine

A day without a latte or a cup of tea or a caffeinated fizzy drink may seem unimaginable for some; however caffeine is a drug, popularly consumed in coffee, tea, soft drinks and, in smaller doses, in chocolate. While we seem to have a love-affair with these products, there's been quite a bit of confusion and even controversy surrounding caffeine lately. In moderation, caffeine is not too bad. However many people become addicted to it as it is a drug and over-indulge - this is when it becomes harmful.

Here are some of the effects it has on your system:

You can feel the effects of caffeine in your system within a few minutes of ingesting it and it stays in your system for many hours. While in your body, caffeine can do the following:

- Inhibit absorption of *adenosine*, which calms the body, which can make you feel alert in the short run, but can cause problems later.
- Inject *adrenaline* into your system, giving you a temporary boost, but possibly making you fatigued and depressed later. If you take more caffeine to counteract these effects, you end up spending the day in an agitated state and might find yourself jumpy and edgy by night.
- Can increase the body's level of *cortisol* (the "stress hormone") which can lead to other health consequences ranging from weight gain and moodiness to heart disease and diabetes.
- Increases *dopamine* levels in your system, acting in a way similar to *amphetamines*, which can make you feel good after taking it, but after it wears off you can feel "low". It can also lead to a physical dependence because of dopamine manipulation.

- Increased levels of cortisol lead to stronger cravings for fat and carbohydrates and cause the body to store fat in the abdomen.
- If caffeine elevates levels of cortisol and other hormones for a temporary boost, after caffeine wears off the body can feel fatigued and feelings of mild to moderate depression can set in. This can make physical activity and exercise more difficult.
- High amounts of caffeine (or stress) can lead to the negative health effects associated with prolonged elevated levels of cortisol. If you ingest high levels of caffeine, you may feel your mood soar and plummet, leaving you craving more caffeine to make it soar again, causing you to lose sleep, suffer health consequences and, of course, feel more stress.

Caffeine withdrawal symptoms can begin as soon as 12 hours after stopping your intake. The symptoms are at their worst after 24 - 48 hours and can last for up to a week. The side effects can include irritability, restlessness, muscle stiffness, difficulty concentrating, headaches, moderate to severe chills and hot spells.

How to Cut out Caffeine

✓ Avoid some of the symptoms by cutting back slowly.
✓ Reduce your caffeine by a half cup per day.
✓ Drink hot water and lemon first thing in the morning to aid the digestive system.
✓ Drink more water.

✓ Drink Green Tea for less caffeine or non
  caffeinated herbal infusions.
✓ Explore the growing world of herbal teas – there
  are some amazing flavours.
✓ Take Guarana and Ginseng if you need an energy
  boost.
✓ Exercise more for extra energy.

Alcohol

Here a few basic facts about alcohol:

- Alcohol is a depressant - this means it can make
  you feel unhappy.
- In whatever form you drink it, alcohol has a similar
  effect on your body. Those who think they will be
  all right if they stick to beer or cider and avoid
  spirits are quite wrong.
- Bubbly drinks (e.g. champagnes, sparkling wines or
  carbonated drinks) will affect you more quickly
  than still drinks because the alcohol in them gets
  into the bloodstream more quickly.
- If you drink on an empty stomach, the alcohol will
  affect you more quickly than if you drink after
  eating a meal.
- As a general rule, the same amount of alcohol will
  affect light people more than heavy people simply
  because it becomes more concentrated in the
  blood.
- The same amount of alcohol will affect a woman
  more than a man regardless of body weight because
  men have higher body water content and so the
  alcohol becomes more diluted in their bodies.

- There is no way of sobering up quickly; black coffee, cold showers and fresh air might make you feel less sleepy but they won't help your body to get rid of the alcohol more quickly.

The alcohol content of drinks is measured in units. There is approximately one unit in each of the following: half a pint of ordinary strength beer; one small glass of wine; one pub measure of spirits. Did you know that one can of super strength lager contains as much alcohol as four pub measures of spirits?

- According to government guidelines, a healthy adult male can drink up to three units and a healthy adult female up to two units per day without harming their health.
- The sensible drinking guidelines for adults apply whether you drink every day or less than this. It is NOT ok to save up units for the weekend. Binge drinking or drinking a lot in one go is very risky and is responsible for most of the problems associated with drinking alcohol.
- Mixing alcohol and other drugs (whether illegal drugs or prescribed medicines) can be dangerous and even fatal.

We are living in a society where alcohol consumption is spiralling out of control - although alcohol consumption has occurred for thousands of years, many of the varied health effects have been discovered fairly recently. Alcohol consumption has health and social consequences via intoxication (drunkenness), dependence (habitual, compulsive and long-term drinking) and other biochemical effects.

In addition to chronic diseases that may affect drinkers after many years of heavy use, alcohol contributes to traumatic outcomes that kill or disable at a relatively young age, resulting in the loss of many years of life to death or disability. There is increasing evidence that besides volume of alcohol, the pattern of the drinking is relevant for the health outcomes. Overall there is a causal relationship between alcohol consumption and more than 60 types of disease and injury.

According to the World Health Organisation, alcohol is estimated to cause about 20-30% worldwide of oesophageal cancer, liver cancer, cirrhosis of the liver, homicide, epilepsy, and motor vehicle accidents. Harmful use of alcohol has a major impact on public health. It is ranked as the fifth leading risk factor for premature death and disability in the world.

In 2002, harmful use of alcohol was estimated to cause about 2.3 million premature deaths worldwide and be responsible for 4.4% of the global disease burden, even after the protective effects of low and moderate alcohol consumption had been considered. Levels, patterns and the social context of drinking differ among regions, nations and communities in studies, but the overall negative health results are clear.

Globally, alcohol consumption has increased in recent decades, with all or most of that increase in developing countries. This increase is often occurring in countries with little tradition of alcohol use on population level and few methods of prevention, control or treatment. The rise in alcohol consumption in developing countries provides ample cause for concern over the possible advent of a matching rise in alcohol-related problems in those regions of the world most at risk.

Drinking a moderate amount of alcohol will not do you any physical or psychological harm. However, for some people, social drinking can lead to heavier drinking, which can cause serious health problems. It is estimated that one in 13 people in the UK are dependent on alcohol (an alcoholic), with several million drinking excessively, to the extent that they are putting their health at risk.

Alcoholism causes many social and health-related problems. If you have an alcohol-related problem, there are many ways in which you can get help to reduce your drinking. There are also many services that can help you give up alcohol altogether.

Many if not the majority of people with alcohol issues are in employment and are more likely to drink over the safe limits than those without jobs. Alcohol is becoming more of an issue in the workplace with an estimated 17 million days lost per year due to alcohol related absenteeism. On top of that there is the cost of mistakes, accidents and under performance.

Smoking

There are actually NO benefits to smoking – if you think it relieves stress, think again. When carbon monoxide and nicotine enter your body, they reduce the supply of oxygen to your brain. Without this oxygen (the fuel of the brain), your brain struggles to function properly, think clearly and concentrate. That, in itself, is extremely stressful!

Around 570 billion cigarettes get smoked around the world a year and it is one of the leading causes of fatal illness. Not only are you putting your own health at risk however; cases of passive smoking related illnesses are significant.

Good reasons to give up smoking

- You will reduce your chances of having a heart attack or stroke.
- You reduce your chances of getting lung cancer, emphysema and other lung diseases.
- You will smell a whole lot nicer and fresher.
- You will climb stairs and walk without getting out of breath.
- You will have fewer wrinkles.
- You will be free of those horrible hacking morning coughs.
- You will have more energy to pursue physical activities.
- You can treat yourself to things with the money you save.

- You will have more control over your life and potentially live longer.
- You will be making your contribution to supporting a healthier environment.

How to Give Up Smoking

✓ Start with some preparation by ensuring that you really do *want* to stop and understanding your reasons for stopping. Are these reasons powerful enough to motivate you when you are faced with those tricky situations? Write down your reasons for stopping.

✓ Ask your doctor for advice. This is especially important if you have health problems or are concerned about issues such as weight gain.

✓ Consider finding yourself a stop-smoking buddy - relatives, work colleagues and friends are a good place to start. Set a date together and you will be able to give each other support.

✓ Tell your family and friends about your intentions. Ask them for their support before you stop and explain that you may not be yourself while experiencing withdrawal. When you reach your stopping date, rely on those that have been most encouraging for support.

✓ Think about starting an exercise programme and a sensible eating plan. Again, speak to your doctor or dietician. Exercise will give you more energy and help you to relax and relieve stress.

✓ You should know what triggers your desire for a cigarette, such as stress, the end of a meal, drinking in a bar, etc. Avoid these triggers while you are trying to quit or if that's not possible, decide how you will deal with the triggers.

✓ Decide what you will do when you experience cravings. As we've discussed, deep breathing, a short walk and keeping yourself busy will help to take your mind off the cravings. Perhaps you can think of other ways. Write them down. Remember: these cravings will only last for 3-5 minutes at a time.

✓ If you have tried stopping before, maybe you came across a stumbling block, which we have discussed, such as finding something to do with your hands. If so, you need to arm yourself with a solution to these foreseeable problems. Get yourself a pen, or stress relief aid to fiddle with, if occupying your hands is a problem.

✓ Be positive and confident you can stop. You have spent time and energy planning how you will deal with the task ahead. You can and will do it if you persevere. Thousands of people around the world every day stop smoking. You can be one of them.

How to be Healthy at Work

✓ Cook a bigger amount on a Sunday, such as veggies and pasta, or chicken and brown rice, and freeze portions to take to work with you for lunch.

✓ Don't skip breakfast! Breakfast kick-starts your metabolism and it's also healthier to eat larger meals earlier in the day because you'll burn them off when you're running around the office.

✓ If you don't have time before work, bring low-fat yogurt (which usually has less sugar than non-fat) and a banana to eat first thing.

✓ Stock your desk area with healthy snacks, so an apple or some raisins are always within reach.

✓ Find the healthiest versions of the snacks you love and bring them to work.

✓ Try one new fruit or vegetable per week. There are plenty of new fruits and vegetables out there for you to try.

✓ Don't completely cut out carbohydrates and fat. Healthy fats, such as those found in nuts (also useful for snacking), and whole grains give you the energy you need to get through the day.

✓ Keep portion size in mind. If you visit the sandwich shop at lunchtime, buy half of a sandwich, or split something with a friend.

✓ Hosting a meeting? Bring some healthy snacks, instead of the usual cakes, biscuits and pastries. Provide fruits and nuts.

✓ Always keep a supply of water handy. Most offices have water coolers, so bring a large glass or thermos or keep a water bottle nearby that you can refill.

✓ Do not eat at your desk. It's a bad habit. Take a lunch break.

Health is a state of complete physical, mental and social well-being and not merely the absence of disease or infirmity

—World Health Organization, 1948

How to Work Wonders with Exercise & Nutrition

✓ Start each day with a hot water and lemon.

✓ Drink herbal and green teas instead of caffeinated drinks.

✓ Aim to drink 2 litres of water a day.

✓ Never skip breakfast.

✓ Snack on fruit, vegetables, nuts and seeds at work.

✓ Keep alcohol consumption within the recommended government limits.

✓ Exercise at least 30 minutes a day.

✓ Practise office exercises.

✓ Wear a pedometer to work.

✓ Take the stairs not the lift.

✓ Encourage walking meetings.

Chapter Three - Communication

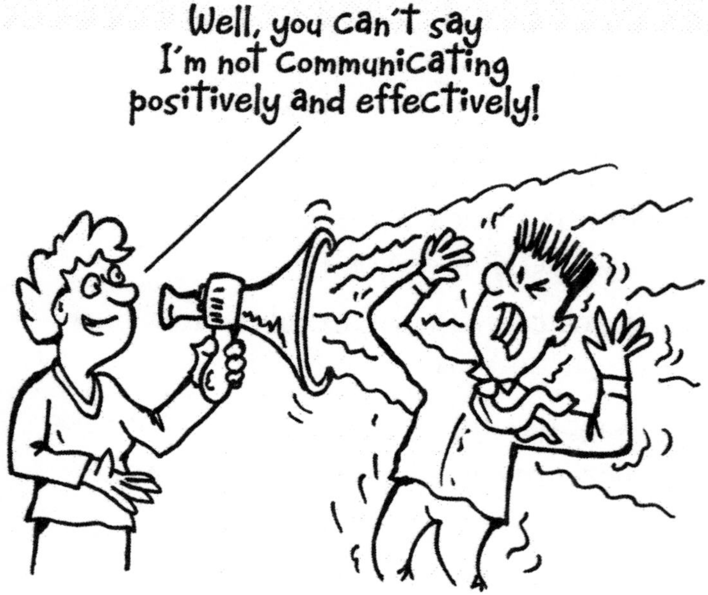

The single biggest problem with communication is the illusion that it has been achieved

George Bernard Shaw

Communication occurs when someone understands you – not just when you speak. One of the biggest dangers with communication is that we can work on the assumption that the other person has understood the message that we are trying to get across.

How many times have we experienced miscommunication through misunderstanding in the work place that has either led to time wasting, deadlines not being met or even conflict?

It is easy to see things from our own perspective, but much more difficult to look at them from another person's, especially when we all have different personalities, backgrounds, ideas and beliefs.

Poor communication in the workplace can lead to a culture of bitching, back stabbing and blame which in turn can also affect our stress levels, especially when we don't understand something or feel that we have been misled. It can also have a very positive effect on morale when it works well and motivates individuals to want to come into work and do a great job.

Modern Communication

The development of communication has provided us, in the last few decades, with a whole new range of media including email, instant messaging, the internet and mobile phones. All of these items undeniably enhance our communication. However, if misused, these gadgets can create issues and pose a problem in the workplace.

It is amazing how many people who sit five feet from each other will actually send each other email rather than speak and I know it is something that I have been guilty of.

The danger we have is that, with more and more consumer-driven technological toys being created, we are starting to *shut out* people in our everyday lives, and the same scenario is occurring in work environments throughout the world. If we really wanted, we now have the ability to go through an entire work day without uttering a word to a single colleague.

Clearly, if we continue to bypass face-to-face communication, our interpersonal skills will suffer as a result. Most human beings need personal interaction, are social creatures and thrive on cultivating and developing relationships with others. Many organisations encourage social interaction between employees and a sense of corporate community can affect staff morale, absenteeism and general overall performance.

So let's explore modern methods of communication in a bit more detail.

Modern Methods of Communication

Email

No doubt about it, email is a very clever and efficient tool. Thanks to the introduction of email, we no longer find memos in our trays, documents can be delivered more quickly and it's easier to relay information to colleagues simultaneously. While all this paper-saving is a dream come true for environmentalists, it doesn't do much to promote interpersonal communication.

Another risky factor about emails is that, if misread, they can easily be misinterpreted. Also, the other one poor communication habit is answering the phone and still continuing to read emails – you can absolutely tell when that happens and it is clear that the person on the other end is not giving you their full attention. It is also poor manners. Just because that person is not in front of you, there is no excuse.

Instant Messaging

IM-ing, as it is now being termed, has become another popular form of communication. While it can be useful if you're trying to reach someone in a hurry, it has also proven to be a large distraction at work. Especially when people use IM to message friends, partners and colleagues simply to chat or to gossip about unrelated work issues, wasting valuable time and energy.

The Internet

One of the most helpful research tools to come along in a long time is hands-down, the internet. From road maps to Christmas cake recipes, you can find any piece of information you need online.

The danger is that it's addictive, even in the workplace, especially now with Facebook and other interactive chat sites becoming available. A great deal of businesses lose valuable productivity time a result of people taking advantage of this forum.

Mobile Phones

By now, pretty much everyone has a mobile phone and quite a few people have two or more. While they are a lifesaver in an emergency, and an effective tool for communication, they can also be a complete pain when people exhibit a lack of mobile phone etiquette.

How many times have you sat in a meeting and somebody's mobile has gone off? Or your colleagues are away from their desk and have forgotten to take their phones with them, thereby resulting in a cacophony of annoying phone rings from Britney Spears to Beethoven's Fifth?

How to Manage Modern Technology

✓ If you can telephone someone, avoid email.
✓ When you are on the phone, do not read your emails at the same time!
✓ Think about the way that you word e-mails to avoid misinterpretation.
✓ Use IM-ing only when absolutely necessary.
✓ Use work internet access for work-related purposes only.
✓ Encourage others to do the same.
✓ If you have to leave your desk, always take your phone with you.
✓ If your mobile rings while working at your desk, speak softly.
✓ Turn your phone off if you are in a meeting.
✓ Remember that face-to-face communication at work is best.

Intelligent and Positive Communication

The key to excellent communication in the workplace is to communicate intelligently and positively. Interestingly enough, a theory of multiple intelligences was developed in 1983 by Dr. Howard Gardner, professor of education at Harvard University.

It suggests that the traditional notion of intelligence, based on IQ testing, is far too limited. Instead, Dr. Gardner proposes eight different intelligences to account for a broader range of human potential in children and adults. These intelligences are:

Linguistic Intelligence

This area has to do with words, spoken or written. People with high verbal-linguistic intelligence display a facility with words and languages. They are typically good at reading, writing, telling stories and memorising words along with dates. They tend to learn best by reading, taking notes, listening to lectures, and discussion and debate.

They are also frequently skilled at explaining, teaching and oration or persuasive speaking. Those with verbal-linguistic intelligence learn foreign languages very easily as they have high verbal memory and recall, and an ability to understand and manipulate syntax and structure. This intelligence is highest in writers, lawyers, philosophers, journalists, politicians, poets, and teachers.

Logical-Mathematical Intelligence

This area has to do with logic, abstractions, reasoning and numbers. It is often assumed that those with this intelligence naturally excel in mathematics, chess, computer-programming and other logical or numerical activities.

A more accurate definition places emphasis on traditional mathematical ability and more reasoning capabilities, abstract patterns of recognition, scientific thinking and investigation, and the ability to perform complex calculations. It correlates strongly with traditional concepts of "intelligence" or IQ. Many scientists, mathematicians, engineers, doctors and economists function on this level of intelligence.

Visual - Spatial Intelligence

This area has to do with vision and spatial judgement. People with strong visual-spatial intelligence are typically very good at visualising and mentally manipulating objects. Those with strong spatial intelligence are often proficient at solving puzzles. They have a strong visual memory and are often artistically inclined.

Those with visual-spatial intelligence also generally have a very good sense of direction and may also have very good hand-eye coordination, although this is normally seen as a characteristic of bodily-kinaesthetic intelligence. Careers that suit those with this intelligence include artists, engineers and architects.

Bodily - Kinaesthetic Intelligence

This area has to do with bodily movement. People who have this intelligence usually learn better by getting up and moving around, and are generally good at physical activities such as sports or dance. They may enjoy acting or performing, and in general they are good at building and making things. They often learn best by doing something physically, rather than reading or hearing about it.

Those with strong bodily-kinaesthetic intelligence seem to use what might be termed muscle memory and they remember things through their body such as verbal memory or images. Careers that suit those with this intelligence include football players, athletes, dancers, actors, surgeons, doctors, builders, and soldiers.

Musical Intelligence

This area has to do with rhythm, music, and hearing. Those who have a high level of musical-rhythmic intelligence display greater sensitivity to sounds, rhythms, absolute pitch and music. They normally have good pitch and may be able to sing, play musical instruments, and compose music.

Since there is a strong auditory component to this intelligence, careers that suit those with this intelligence include instrumentalists, singers, conductors, disc-jockeys, orators, writers and composers.

Interpersonal Intelligence

This area has to do with interaction with others. People who have a high interpersonal intelligence tend to be extroverts, characterised by their sensitivity to others' moods, feelings, temperaments and motivations, and their ability to cooperate in order to work as part of a group.

They communicate effectively and empathise easily with others, and may be either leaders or followers. They typically learn best by working with others and often enjoy discussion and debate. Careers that suit those with this intelligence include politicians, teachers, managers and social workers.

Intrapersonal Intelligence

This area has to do with introspective and self-reflective capacities. They are usually highly self-aware and capable of understanding their own emotions, goals and motivations. They often have an affinity for thought-based pursuits such as philosophy. They learn best when allowed to concentrate on the subject by themselves.

There is often a high level of perfectionism associated with this intelligence. Careers that suit those with this intelligence include philosophers, psychologists, theologians, writers and scientists.

Naturalist Intelligence

This area has to do with nature, nurturing and relating information to one's natural surroundings. Those with it are said to have greater sensitivity to nature and their place within it, the ability to nurture and grow things, and greater ease in caring for, taming and interacting with animals. They may also be able to discern changes in the weather or similar fluctuations in their natural surroundings. Recognising and classifying things are at the core of a *naturalist*.

They must connect a new experience with prior knowledge to truly learn something new. Naturalists learn best when the subject involves collecting and analysing, or is closely related to something prominent in nature; they also don't enjoy learning unfamiliar or seemingly useless subjects with little or no connections to nature. It is advised that naturalistic learners would learn more through being outside or working in a kinaesthetic way. Careers that suit those with this intelligence include vets, environmentalists, scientists, gardeners and farmers.

Dr. Gardner believes that our schools and culture focus most of their attention on linguistic and logical-mathematical intelligence. We esteem the highly articulate or logical people of our culture. However, Dr. Gardner says that we should also place equal attention on individuals who show gifts in the other intelligences: the artists, architects, musicians, naturalists, designers, dancers, therapists, entrepreneurs and others who enrich the world in which we live.

Unfortunately, many children who have these gifts don't receive much reinforcement for them in school. Many of these children, in fact, end up being labelled "learning disabled", are charged with ADD (attention deficit disorder) or are simply deemed as underachievers, when their unique ways of thinking and learning aren't addressed by a heavily linguistic or logical-mathematical classroom.

The theory of multiple intelligences proposes a major transformation in the way our schools are run. It suggests that teachers be trained to present their lessons in a wide variety of ways using music, cooperative learning, art activities, role play, multimedia, field trips, inner reflection, and much more.

The two areas of communication that are heavily linked to intelligence in the work place and indeed anywhere are *intrapersonal* and *interpersonal* communication. Intrapersonal communication is about the communication that you have with yourself, it is the little voice inside your head that talks to you and shapes your perception of the world around you. Interpersonal communication is about the way in which you communicate and interact with others. I would like to tackle each of these two areas separately.

Intrapersonal Communication

Many people believe that the art of communication is all about how we communicate with others. This is a great fallacy, because the way in which you communicate with yourself is the first step to positive and effective communication.

I believe we really underestimate our potential to improve our communication because we simply do not take the time to listen to the little voice inside our heads and what we are saying to ourselves consciously and subconsciously. According to some experts, we communicate with ourselves over 50,000 times a day and our self-talk is capable of using hundreds of words per minute to communicate with ourselves. That is clearly a lot of dialogue to listen to.

As I outlined in Chapter One with regards to attitude, what we think and what we allow our internal voice to programme us with, we act upon. Dennis Waitley, who wrote *The Psychology of Winning* (a book I have been carrying around with me for the last twenty years) said "What the mind dwells upon, the body acts upon".

Our reality is our perception and our perception is our reality. In the book *Change your Life, Change your Thinking* by Brian Tracy it is highlighted that some of the most successful communicators are those who are very aware of their thoughts and self-talk and take control of the way in which they communicate with themselves. So this really is the first area that needs addressing if you want to communicate more successfully at work and with those around you.

Positive Self Speak

Take a good listen to your personal vocabulary – How do you speak to yourself? Vocabulary is something we very rarely pay conscious attention to, yet it can give away a host of information about us to the perceptive listener.

Like appearance, vocabulary and speech form part of that important "first impression" we make on other people. While the tone and timbre of our voices creates either a pleasing or grating effect on the listener, our choice of words conveys our attitude and emotional stance. There is a very interesting relationship between vocabulary and attitude.

When you describe an emotional state or use words to express an emotion directly, you reinforce that emotion. If, for example, you say, "Damn!" when you make a mistake, you reinforce the anger you feel about the mistake. If instead however you say "Oops!" you're conveying to your subconscious mind that the mistake was minor, something not worth getting too excited about.

Modifying your vocabulary is one way to reduce the number of times you experience strong stressful emotions like anger. The same principle applies to positive emotions.

Have you ever asked someone how they are and they answered, *"Not too bad, thanks."* What if they'd answered instead, *"*I'm excellent!" or "I'm feeling great. Thanks for asking!" How would that affect the person's attitude towards his or her life?

Anthony Robbins, in his best-selling book *Awaken the Giant Within*, suggests writing a list of words you'd like to change in both positive and negative situations. For example, you might replace a lukewarm positive word like "nice" with "great", and change a negative word like "depressed" to "less energetic". He also advises getting leverage on yourself by asking three friends to pull you up when you slip back into old language patterns.

Positive self-talk is a great way to improve your energy levels. Most people know it by its more straightforward name of affirmations. But you need something a bit more focused than the traditional: "Every day in every way, I'm getting better and better". When you are using positive self-talk to improve your energy levels you need to make sure that your subconscious is in no doubt as to what you are talking about.

There are a great many books that have been written in the self-improvement genre on positive affirmations and if you do not think that you are able to devise your own, then you should have no trouble in finding something at your local bookshop.

When you are doing the affirmations, make sure that you have a very clear goal in mind as to what you are trying to achieve. If your wording is too vague or you are not focused enough on what you are trying to achieve, then you may not get the results that you are looking for. For instance if you are trying to encourage yourself to go for a good long walk every day, there is no point in making a vague statement to yourself such as "I would like to get out and about more".

You need to be very clear as to what you are trying to encourage yourself to do. A much more concise affirmation would be, "I go for a walk every day in the park when I get back from work and it is very enjoyable". This way, the mind is left in no doubt as to what you are trying to achieve and what is required of it.

When you are making affirmations to improve your energy levels, it is very important that all of your affirmations are not only in the present tense, but are also in the positive. It is very important to keep the affirmations in the positive as the subconscious mind is not able to process a negative very well.

Rather than trying to get the subconscious mind to extract a positive action from a negative affirmation, it is much easier to put the affirmation in the positive in the first place. A good example of this would be for someone who is trying to lose weight using affirmations. If the affirmation is in the negative as in this text, "I will not eat fast food any more" then it is very difficult for the subconscious mind to process.

The mind not only has to process the negative as in what you are not going to do, i.e. eat fast food, it also has to then decide, subconsciously, what it is actually supposed to be doing instead, i.e. eating well, which in itself is not a clearly defined concept. But if you put the affirmation in a positive sense, "I am eating fresh fruit and salad every day" then it is very clear what is required of the mind and it is much easier to process this into action.

When you are doing positive self-talk, it is necessary to do it on a regular and consistent basis. The effects are usually cumulative and you should find that the more you do it, the more effective it is in helping you to build up your energy levels and to improve the way in which you live. This is partly due to the effect of saying something over and over again, but also, if your mind is used to you using affirmations and to processing them into action, then it is more likely to be able to process new affirmations as it is just following on in the pattern of the previous, albeit different, affirmations that you have used in the past. This way you can gain the benefits more quickly but you still need to use repetitions of the positive self-talk until you have achieved the right results.

One way in which you can use this to build your energy levels is to use affirmations such as *"I am happy and always have enough energy to enjoy my work throughout the day"*. This places the affirmation in the positive and also in the present. It also states very clearly what you are not only hoping to achieve, but what is actually happening.

Using positive self-talk can not only help to improve your energy directly but it can also help you to achieve other ways of improving your energy levels, such as exercising and improving your diet. Exercising and eating well can have really beneficial effects on your energy levels, but can be very hard for many people to get used to.

Using positive affirmations can really help you to change the way that you eat and also make it much easier for you to get used to doing an exercise programme. It is important not to limit the way that you use affirmations to just the direct benefit that you are looking for. If you try to look at all the different ways that you can use affirmations, you will find a great many ways in which they can benefit you.

The most important thing is to consciously and regularly listen to yourself and the words that you are using to condition your thoughts which will in turn trigger your emotions which shape your actions which ultimately define your world!

Just a Thought

Yesterday I had a thought.
That thought became an emotion,
That emotion turned into words,
The words fuelled action,
The actions became a habit.
My habits are my Character,
My Character defines my destiny.
Today, therefore,
I'll think about my thoughts a little more.

Self - Confidence

Self-esteem and self-confidence are a really important part of intrapersonal communication and being able to communicate positively. We looked at the concept of internal and external referencing in Chapter One and the importance of being able to be balanced in your ability to *internally* and *externally* reference yourself.

There are many ways to develop self confidence and what works for some may not work for another. However, here are few suggestions:

How to Improve Your Confidence

✓ Trust Yourself
This is the real key to self confidence. It is about

believing in yourself and trusting your own views and opinions. This, at times, can be difficult, especially if you have a tendency to listen to others and benchmark yourself against what they think of you. This is, however, very dangerous and the ability to be able to establish your own inner benchmark to success is essential.

✓ Like Yourself

If there is something about yourself that you do not like then you may be able to change it. However consider this:

> *Grant me the serenity*
> *to accept the things I cannot change;*
> *courage to change the things I can;*
> *and wisdom to know the difference.*
> —*Reinhold Niebuhr*

Every human being has the ability to take control and make positive changes. Other people can try and stop you, but only if you let them. When you look in the mirror, be proud of the person that you see, knowing that you do the best you can.

✓ Listen to Yourself

Tell yourself that you are confident and believe in yourself. Focus on your strengths and the positive aspects of your character and set about developing the area that you have for potential.

✓ Develop Good Posture

The way a person carries themselves tells a story. People with slumped shoulders and lethargic movements display a lack of self confidence. They aren't enthusiastic about what they're doing and they don't consider themselves important. By practising good posture, you'll automatically feel more confident. Stand up straight, keep your head up, and make eye contact. You'll make a positive impression on others and instantly feel more alert and empowered.

✓ Motivate Yourself

One of the best ways to build confidence is listening to a motivational speech. There are some great CDs out there. You can even write your own. Write a 30-60 second speech that highlights your strengths and goals. Then recite it in front of the mirror aloud (or inside your head if you prefer) whenever you need a confidence boost.

✓ Develop an Attitude of Gratitude

Be grateful for what you have. Set aside time each day to mentally list everything you have to be grateful for. Recall your past successes, unique skills, loving relationships, and positive momentum. You'll be amazed how much you have going for you and motivated to take that next step towards success.

✓ Compliment Other People

When we think negatively about ourselves, we often project that feeling on to others in the form of insults and gossip. To break this cycle of negativity, get in the habit of praising other people. Refuse to engage in backstabbing office gossip and make an effort to compliment those around you. In the process, you'll become well liked and, by looking for the best in others, you indirectly bring out the best in yourself.

✓ Sit in the Front Row

In meetings and public assemblies around the world, people constantly strive to sit at the back of the room. Most people prefer the back because they're afraid of being noticed. This reflects a lack of self-confidence. By deciding to sit in the front row, you can get over this irrational fear and build your self-confidence. You'll also be more visible to the important people talking from the front of the room.

✓ Speak Up

During group discussions and meetings at work, many people never speak up because they're afraid that people will judge them for saying something stupid. This fear isn't really justified. Generally, people are much more accepting than we imagine. In fact, most people are dealing with the exact same fears. By making an effort to speak up at least once in every group discussion, you'll become a better public speaker, more confident in your own thoughts, and recognised as a leader by your peers.

✓ Exercise

Along the same lines as personal appearance, physical fitness has a huge effect on self confidence. If you're out of shape, you'll feel insecure, unattractive, and less energetic. By working out, you improve your physical appearance, energise yourself, and accomplish something positive. Having the discipline to work out not only makes you feel better, it creates positive momentum that you can build on for the rest of the day.

✓ Walk Faster

One of the easiest ways to tell how a person feels about themselves is to examine their walk. Is it slow? Tired? Painful? Or is it energetic and purposeful? People with confidence walk quickly. They have places to go, people to see, and important work to do. Even if you aren't in a hurry, you can increase your self-confidence by putting some pep in your step. Walking 25% faster will make you look and feel more energised and confident.

✓ Look Outwards

Too often we get caught up in our own desires. We focus too much on ourselves and not enough on the needs of other people. If you stop thinking about yourself and concentrate on the contribution you're making to the rest of the world, you won't worry as much about you own flaws. This will increase self-confidence and allow you to contribute with maximum efficiency. The more you contribute to the world, the more you'll be rewarded with personal success and recognition.

Developing a sense of self awareness and understanding yourself will help to develop your *Intrapersonal* communication skills and this is the first step to becoming a better communicator.

Interpersonal Communication

Interpersonal communication is essentially how we communicate with others. This can encompass verbal, written and nonverbal forms of communication. The term is usually applied to spoken communication that takes place between two or more individuals on a personal, face-to-face level.

There are many ways that we communicate in the workplace, informal chats, staff meetings, formal project discussions, employee performance reviews, learning and development activities to name a few. Interpersonal communication with those outside of the business environment can take a variety of forms as well, including client meetings, employment interviews or sales visits.

We are all unique and the way in which we communicate can vary quite a bit. Through our lifetime, we define different definitions and interpretations of language and expression. We also work in far more diverse multicultural environments. The celebration of diversity in organisations is recognised as something that is very positive; however, it also has its challenges.

Over the past few years, I have been working with some very diverse organisations in both the private and public sector. As a consultant for the United Nations, I am exposed to a range of cultures and communication styles which have been a wonderful education.

Respect and appreciation of diversity in people is so positive and brings a whole range of possibilities, opportunities and experience to organisations. The trick is to try to see things from other people's perspective in order to broaden your ability and your range of communication.

Understanding Communication

Professor Albert Mehrabian pioneered the understanding of communications since the 1960s. Aside from his many and various other fascinating works, Mehrabian established this classic statistic for the effectiveness of face to face communication. His findings concluded the following:

- 7% of meaning is in the words that are spoken.
- 38% of meaning is your tone of voice.
- 55% of meaning is non verbal communication.

Mehrabian's model has become one of the most widely referenced statistics in communications. The theory is particularly useful in explaining the importance of meaning, as distinct from words.

The value of Mehrabian's theory relates to communications where emotional content is significant, and the need to understand it properly is essential to mitigate the risk of misunderstandings. This is so important in the workplace, where motivation and attitude have a crucial effect on outcomes.

Understanding the difference between words and meaning is a vital capability for effective communications and relationships.

The understanding of how to convey when speaking and interpret when listening will always be essential for effective communication, management and relationships.

Transferring Mehrabian's findings to emails and telephone conversations, for example, is simply to say that greater care needs to be taken in the use of language and expression, because the visual channel does not exist.

It is fair to say that email and other written communications are limited to conveying words alone. The way that the words are said cannot be conveyed, and facial expression cannot be conveyed at all. Mehrabian provides us with a reference point as to why written communications, particularly quick, reduced emails and memos, so often result in confusion or cause offence.

Modern text-based communications allow inclusion of simple iconic facial expressions (smileys, and other emotional symbols), which further proves the significance of, and natural demand for, non-verbal signs within communications.

Telephone communication can convey words and the way that the words are said, but no facial expression. Mehrabian's model provides clues as to why telephone communications are less successful and reliable for sensitive or emotional issues.

118

Video-conferencing communications are not as reliable as genuine face-to-face communications because of the intermittent transfer of images, which is, of course, incapable of conveying accurate non-verbal signals. Video conferencing offers a massive benefit for modern organisation development and cooperation. Be aware of its vulnerabilities, and use it wherever it's appropriate, because it is a great system.

Understanding Your Communication Style

Good communication skills require a high level of self-awareness. Understanding your personal style of communicating will go a long way toward helping you to create good and lasting impressions on others. By becoming more aware of how others perceive you, you can adapt more readily to their styles of communicating.

This does not mean you have to be a chameleon, changing with every personality you meet. Instead, you can make another person more comfortable with you by selecting and emphasising certain behaviours that fit within your personality and resonate with another.

You may well be familiar with the term psychometrics – from the Latin term it means *measurement of the mind.*

Many organisations use a range of psychometrics as part of their recruitment process or staff development, as these tests can give a insight into individuals' personalities, behaviours and preferred style of communication. The best that I have come across recently is *Facet 5* which looks at an individual's behaviour, motivation, attitudes, aspirations and emotionality. It speaks plain language with no jargon or psychobabble and has many uses in many languages. There are however many on the market and they are extremely useful tools in terms of developing self awareness and improving individuals' ability to develop their potential.

Assertive Communication

Assertive communication is an excellent interpersonal skill to develop. It is the ability to express your thoughts and opinions while respecting the thoughts and opinions of the other person. Assertive communication is appropriately direct, open and honest, and clarifies your needs to the other person. Assertiveness is a skill that can be learned. People who have mastered the skill of assertiveness are able to greatly reduce the level of interpersonal conflict in their lives and significantly reduce a major source of stress.

Take a look at these contrasting styles and examine how these may relate to you – be really honest with yourself.

Aggressive Communication

Beliefs

- Everyone should be like me.

- I am never wrong.
- I've got rights, but you don't.

Communication Style

- Closed-minded.
- Poor listener.
- Has difficulty seeing the other person's point of view.
- Interrupts.
- Monopolising conversations.

Characteristics

- Achieves goals, often at others' expense.
- Domineering, bullying.
- Patronising.
- Condescending, sarcastic.

Behaviour

- Puts others down.
- Doesn't ever think they are wrong.
- Bossy.
- Moves into people's space, overpowers.
- Easily jumps on others and pushes people around.
- Know-it-all attitude.
- Doesn't show appreciation.

Nonverbal Communication

- Points, shakes finger.
- Frowns.

- Squints eyes critically.
- Glares.
- Stares.
- Rigid posture.
- Critical, loud, yelling tone of voice.
- Fast, clipped speech.

Verbal Communication

- You must /should.
- Don't ask why - Just do it.
- General verbal abuse.

Confrontation and Problem Solving

- Must win arguments, threatens, attacks.
- Operates from win/lose position.

Effects

- Provokes counter-aggression, alienation from others, ill health.
- Wastes time and energy over-supervising others
- Pays high price in human relationships.
- Fosters resistance, defiance, sabotaging, striking back, forming alliances, lying, covering up.
- Forces compliance with resentment.

Passive Communicators

Beliefs

- Don't express your true feelings.
- Don't make waves.

- Don't disagree.
- Others have more rights than I do.

Communication Style

- Indirect.
- Always agrees.
- Doesn't speak up.
- Hesitant.

Characteristics

- Apologetic, self-conscious.
- Trusts others, but not self.
- Doesn't express own wants and feelings.
- Allows others to make decisions for self.
- Doesn't get what he or she wants.

Behaviours

- Sighs a lot.
- Tries to sit on both sides of the fence to avoid conflict.
- Clams up when feeling treated unfairly.
- Asks permission unnecessarily.
- Complains instead of taking action.
- Lets others make choices.
- Has difficulty implementing plans.
- Self-effacing.
- Fidgets.
- Nods head often; comes across as pleading.
- Lack of facial animation.
- Slumped posture.
- Fast, when anxious; slow, hesitant, when doubtful.

Verbal Communication

- You could/should do it.
- You have more experience than I do.
- I can't /I'm afraid.
- This is probably wrong, but ….
- I'll try ….

Confrontation and Problem Solving

- Avoids, ignores, leaves, postpones.
- Withdraws, is sullen and silent.
- Agrees externally, while disagreeing internally.
- Expends energy to avoid conflicts that are anxiety-provoking.
- Spends too much time asking for advice, supervision.
- Agrees too often.

Effects

- Gives up being him or herself.
- Builds dependency relationships.
- Doesn't know where he or she stands.
- Slowly loses self-esteem.
- Promotes others' causes.
- Is not well-liked.

How to Communicate Assertively

Beliefs

- Believe in yourself and other people.
- Know that assertiveness doesn't mean you always

win, but that you handled the situation as effectively as possible.

- You have rights and so do others.

Communication Style

- Be an effective and active listener.
- State limits and expectations.
- Observe without labelling or judging.
- Express yourself directly, honestly, and as soon as possible.
- Be aware of others' feelings.

Characteristics

- Non-judgmental.
- Trust yourself and others.
- Be confident.
- Be self-aware.
- Be open, flexible, versatile.
- Be playful with an appropriate sense of humour.
- Be decisive.
- Be proactive and take the initiative.

Behaviour

- Operate from choice.
- Know what is needed and develop a plan to get it.
- Be action-oriented.
- Be firm and fair.
- Be realistic about your expectations.
- Be consistent and reliable.
- Be trustworthy.

Nonverbal Communication

- Use open and natural gestures.
- Be attentive with interested facial expressions.
- Use direct eye contact.
- Adopt a confident and relaxed posture.
- Use appropriate volume and pace of speech.

Verbal Communication Examples

- I choose to ….
- What are my options?
- What are your views?
- What alternatives do we have?

Confrontation and Problem Solving

- Negotiate, bargain, trade off, compromise.
- Confront problems at the time they happen.
- Don't let negative feelings build up.

Effects and Benefits

- Increased self-esteem and self-confidence.
- Increased self-esteem of others.
- Feel motivated and understood.
- Others will know where they stand.
- Others will respect you.

So, assertive communication is one of the best ways to get your message across.

Listening Skills

Listening and understanding what others communicate to us is the most important part of successful interaction and vice versa. When a person decides to communicate with another person, they do so to fulfil a need. The person wants something, feels discomfort, has feelings or thoughts about something. In deciding to communicate, the person selects the method or code which they believe will effectively deliver the message to the other person. The code used to send the message can be either verbal or nonverbal. When the other person receives the coded message, they go through the process of decoding or interpreting it into understanding and meaning. Effective communication exists between two people when the receiver interprets and understands the sender's message in the same way the sender intended it. Simple, you may think!

We were given two ears but only one mouth, because listening is twice as hard as talking.

What are the Challenges to Listening?

- Being preoccupied and not listening 100% because your internal voice is having a little chat with you.
- Being so interested in what you have to say that you are listening mainly for a gap so that you can jump in with your bit.

- Formulating and listening to your own rebuttal that you are going to respond with.
- Listening to your own personal beliefs about what is being said.
- Evaluating and making judgements about the speaker or the message.
- Not asking for clarification when you know that you do not understand.

The Three Basic Listening Modes

- **Competitive** or **Combative Listening** happens when we are more interested in promoting our own point of view than in understanding or exploring someone else's view. We either listen for openings to take the floor, or for flaws or weak points we can attack. As we pretend to pay attention we are impatiently waiting for an opening, or internally formulating our rebuttal and planning our devastating comeback that will destroy their argument and make us the victor.
- **In Passive** or **Attentive Listening** we are genuinely interested in hearing and understanding the other person's point of view. We are attentive and passively listen. We assume that we heard and understand correctly, but stay passive and do not verify it.
- **Active** or **Reflective Listening** is the single most useful and important listening skill. In active listening, we are also genuinely interested in understanding what the other person is thinking, feeling, wanting or what the message means, and

we are active in checking out our understanding before we respond with our own new message. We restate or paraphrase our understanding of their message and reflect it back to the sender for verification. This verification or feedback process is what distinguishes active listening and makes it effective.

Levels of Communication

Listening effectively is difficult, because people vary in their communication skills and in how clearly they express themselves, and often have different needs, wants and purposes for interacting. The different types of interaction or levels of communication also adds to the difficulty. The four different types or levels are:

- Clichés
- Facts
- Thoughts and beliefs
- Feelings and emotions

As a listener, we attend to the level that we think is most important. Failing to recognise the level most relevant and important to the speaker, can lead to a kind of *crossed wires* where the two people are not on the same wavelength. The purpose of the contact and the nature of our relationship with the person will usually determine what level or levels are appropriate and important for the particular interaction. If we don't address the appropriate elements, we will not be very effective, and can actually make the situation worse.

For example: if your wife is telling you about her hurt feelings and you focus on the facts of the situation and don't acknowledge her feelings, she will likely become even more upset.

There is a real distinction between merely *hearing the words* and really listening for the message. When we listen effectively we understand what the person is thinking and/or feeling from the other person's own perspective. It is as if we were standing in the other person's shoes, seeing through his/her eyes and listening through the person's ears. Our own viewpoint may be different and we may not necessarily agree with the person, but as we listen, we understand from the other's perspective. To listen effectively, we must be actively involved in the communication process, and not just listening passively.

We all act and respond on the basis of our under- standing, and too often there is a misunderstanding that neither of us is aware of. With active listening, if a misunderstanding has occurred, it will be known immediately, and the communication can be clarified before any further misunderstanding occurs.

Several other possible benefits occur with active listening:

- Sometimes a person just needs to be heard and acknowledged before the person is willing to consider an alternative or soften his/her position.

- It is often easier for a person to listen to and consider the other's position when that person knows the other is listening and considering his/her position.
- It helps people to spot the flaws in their reasoning when they hear it played back without criticism.
- It also helps identify areas of agreement so the areas of disagreement are put in perspective and are diminished rather than magnified.
- Reflecting back what we hear each other say helps give each a chance to become aware of the different levels that are going on below the surface. This helps to bring things into the open where they can be more readily resolved.
- If we accurately understand the other person's view, we can be more effective in helping the person see the flaws in his/her position.
- If we listen so we can accurately understand the other's view, we can also be more effective in discovering the flaws in our own position.

How to Be a Good Listener

✓ Give yourself permission to listen and give 100% attention by telling the little voice inside your head to shut up so that you can focus.

✓ Use eye contact and *listening* body language. Avoid looking at your watch or at other people or activities around the room. Face and lean toward the speaker and nod your head, as it is appropriate. Be careful about crossing your arms and appearing closed or critical.

✓ Be empathic and nonjudgmental. You can be

accepting and respectful of the person and their feelings and beliefs without invalidating or giving up your own position, or without agreeing with the accuracy and validity of their view.

✓ Paraphrase and use your own words in verbalising your understanding of the message. Parroting back the words verbatim is annoying and does not ensure accurate understanding of the message.

✓ Don't respond to just the meaning of the words, look for the feelings or intent beyond the words. The dictionary or surface meaning of the words or code used by the sender is not the message.

✓ Inhibit your impulse to immediately answer questions. The code may be in the form of a question. Sometimes people ask questions when they really want to express themselves and are not open to hearing an answer.

✓ Know when to quit using active listening. Once you accurately understand the sender's message, it may be appropriate to respond with your own message. Don't use active listening to hide and avoid revealing your own position.

✓ If you are confused and know you do not understand, either tell the person you don't understand and ask him/her to say it another way, or use your best guess. If you are incorrect, the person will realise it and will likely attempt to correct your misunderstanding.

Positive Communication

Positive communication is really important in the workplace in order to create a happy working environment. We all have responsibility for the way that we come into work and in Chapter One we talked about NAGs – Negative Attitude Germs. Try to be the work radiator, not the drain.

It is very easy to blame everyone else and everything else for anything that you may feel. It is also easy to let other people get on your nerves and wind you up, but *only* if you let them. However, if you take responsibility, and set a positive example, it will be positive step in the right direction of working wonders with Communication at work.

> *Communication leads to community, that is, to understanding, intimacy and mutual valuing.*
>
> —*Rollo May*

How to Work Wonders with Communication

- ✓ Be a radiator and communicate positively.
- ✓ Be self-aware and emotionally intelligent.
- ✓ Understand your communication style.
- ✓ Appreciate that other people have different strengths and weaknesses.
- ✓ Be supportive to those around you.
- ✓ Use humour appropriately in the workplace.
- ✓ Respect and celebrate diversity.
- ✓ Actively listen and focus.
- ✓ Two ears, one mouth - use them in that quantity.
- ✓ Be an assertive communicator.
- ✓ Choose win-win outcomes.
- ✓ If in doubt, check your understanding.
- ✓ Encourage feedback about your communication.
- ✓ Use positive non-verbal communication.
- ✓ Smile – it is the universal currency in communication.

Chapter Four
Stress Management

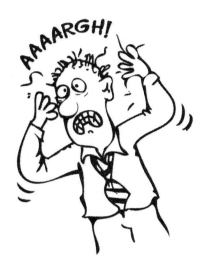

Adopting the right attitude can convert a negative stress into a positive one

Hans Selye

A woman accompanied her husband to the doctor's office because he had been suffering with headaches and lack of sleep; he seemed especially irritable and generally out of sorts. After the man had completed his check up, the doctor called his wife into his office alone.

He told her: "Your husband is suffering from high levels of stress. If you don't do the following, your husband will surely die."

"What can I do to help him?" asked his wife.

The doctor continued, "To help reduce his stress each morning you must get up before him and fix him a healthy breakfast. Be pleasant at all times. Prepare him a nutritious packed lunch. When he comes home from work greet him with a happy smile, do not burden him with chores; do not discuss your problems with him, as it will only make his stress worse. There must be absolutely no nagging. You must also give your husband any amount of affection he requires, whenever he demands. If you can do this for the next ten months to a year, I think it will help to reduce his stress levels and he could well regain his health completely."

On the way home, the concerned husband asked his wife, "What did the doctor say to you?"

To which his wife responded, "He said it looks like you are going to die."

Stress in the Modern World

There is, however, a very dark side of stress with more and more people being affected every single day.

In 2006, 175 million working days were lost due to illness and absenteeism. Stress is believed to trigger 70% of visits to doctors and 85% of serious illnesses according to the Health and Safety Executive (HSE) which is a non-departmental body responsible for the encouragement, regulation and enforcement of workplace health, safety and welfare.

According to the American Psychological Association (APA), one-third of Americans are living with extreme stress and nearly half of Americans believe that their stress levels have increased over the past five years.

A little bit of pressure can be productive, give you motivation, and help you to perform better at something. However, too much pressure or prolonged pressure can lead to stress, which is unhealthy for the mind and body. Everyone reacts differently to stress, and some people may have a higher threshold than others. Too much stress often leads to physical, mental and emotional problems.

Anxiety and depression are the most common mental health problems, and the majority of cases are caused by stress. Research by mental health charities also suggests that a quarter of the population will have a mental health problem at some point in their lives.

What is Stress?

Stress is your body's way of responding to any kind of demand or pressure. It can be caused by both positive and negative experiences. When people feel stressed by something going on around them, their bodies react by releasing certain chemicals into the bloodstream.

These chemicals give people more energy and strength, which can be a good thing if their stress is caused by physical danger. This, however, can also be a bad thing, if their stress is in response to something emotional and there is no outlet for this extra energy and strength.

Many different things can cause stress. Identifying what may be causing you stress is often the first step in learning how to cope. Some of the most common sources of stress are:

Survival Stress

You may have heard the phrase "fight or flight"; this is a common response to danger in all people and animals. When you are afraid that someone or something may be trying to hurt you, your body naturally responds with a burst of energy so that you will be better able to survive the dangerous situation (fight) or escape it altogether (flight).

Internal Stress

Have you ever worried about things that have happened that you can do nothing about or tried to gaze into a crystal ball and worried about things imagined in the future that you have absolutely no control over? We all do, I am sure, from time to time. This is internal stress and it is one of the most important kinds of stress to understand and manage. Internal stress is when people make themselves stressed.

Some people become addicted to stress and the kind of hurried, tense, lifestyle that results from being under stress. They even look for stressful situations and feel stressed about things that aren't stressful. This, for some people, like coffee, is a stimulant that acts as false energy and motivation.

Environmental Stress

This is a response to things around you that cause stress, such as noise, crowding and pressure from work or family. Identifying these environmental stresses and learning to avoid them or deal with them will help lower your stress level.

Fatigue and Overwork

This kind of stress builds up over a long time and can take a hard toll on your body. It can be caused by working too much or too hard. It can also be caused by not knowing how to manage your time well or how to take time out for rest and relaxation. This can be one of the hardest kinds of stress to avoid because many people feel this is out of their control.

Stress can affect both your body and your mind. People under large amounts of stress can become tired, sick, and unable to concentrate or think clearly. Sometimes, stress can even trigger severe depression and mental breakdowns.

Stress at Work

In our fast-paced society, the term *stress-related burnout* seems to almost go with the territory. It certainly seems to be an ever-present reality. Just-in-time development, instantaneous information from around the world, mobile communication and a whole swarm of other progressive technologies are a great benefit. However, in conjunction, these reap earlier deadlines and increased pressure.

Clearly, the rising figures of stress-related illness are very concerning for many organisations who keep the interest and well being of their people at the heart of their business. Many employers attempt to provide a stress-free work environment and recognise where it is becoming a problem for staff, and take action to reduce it.

Stress in the workplace reduces productivity, increases management pressures, and makes people ill in many ways, evidence of which is worryingly still increasing. Stress at work also provides a serious risk of litigation for all employers and organisations, carrying significant liabilities for damages, bad publicity and loss of reputation.

Dealing with stress-related claims also consumes vast amounts of management time. So there are clearly strong economic and financial reasons for organisations to manage and reduce stress at work, aside from the obvious humanitarian and ethical considerations.

Lord Philip Hunt OBE, Parliamentary Under-Secretary of State has indeed emphasised the strong benefits to individuals, organisations and society who effectively manage stress at work.

He gave full Government backing for the *Health and Safety Executive (HSE) - Management Standards for Work-Related Stress*, at a conference arranged to mark National Stress Awareness Day in 2005.

In 2005, Lord Hunt stressed: "Over half a million people in the UK currently experience stress at a level they believe is making them ill, and this costs society over £3.7 billion per year. The Government is committed to tackling this issue."

The *Strategy for the Health and Wellbeing of Working Age People* was introduced and, as a result, the Government now attaches great importance to the health and wellbeing of working age people.

Management Standards

The *Management Standards* define the characteristics, or culture, of an organisation where the risks from work-related stress are being effectively managed and controlled.

The *Management Standards* cover six key areas of work design that, if not properly managed, are associated with poor health and wellbeing, lower productivity and increased sickness absence. In other words, the six *Management Standards* cover the primary sources of stress at work. These are:

Demands

This includes issues such as workload, work patterns and the work environment.

The Standard is that employees indicate that they are able to cope with the demands of their jobs; and systems are in place locally to respond to any individual concerns.

- The organisation provides employees with adequate and achievable demands in relation to the agreed hours of work.
- People's skills and abilities are matched to the job demands.

- Jobs are designed to be within the capabilities of employees.
- Employees' concerns about their work environment are addressed.

Control

This is how much say the person has in the way they do their work.

The Standard is that employees indicate that they are able to have a say about the way they do their work and systems are in place locally to respond to any individual concerns.

- Where possible, employees have control over their pace of work.
- Employees are encouraged to use their skills and initiative to do their work.
- Where possible, employees are encouraged to develop new skills to help them undertake new and challenging pieces of work.
- The organisation encourages employees to develop their skills
- Employees have a say over when breaks can be taken.
- Employees are consulted over their work patterns.

Support

This includes the encouragement, sponsorship and resources provided by the organisation, line management and colleagues. Employees indicate that they receive adequate information and support from their colleagues and superiors and systems are in place locally to respond to any individual concerns.

- The organisation has policies and procedures to adequately support employees.
- Systems are in place to enable and encourage managers to support their staff.
- Systems are in place to enable and encourage employees to support their colleagues.
- Employees know what support is available and how and when to access it.
- Employees know how to access the required resources to do their job.
- Employees receive regular and constructive feedback.

Relationships

This includes promoting positive working to avoid conflict, and dealing with unacceptable behaviour. Employees indicate that they are not subjected to unacceptable behaviours (for example, bullying at work) and systems are in place locally to respond to any individual concerns.

- The organisation promotes positive behaviours at work to avoid conflict and ensure fairness.
- Employees share information relevant to their work.
- The organisation has agreed policies and procedures to prevent or resolve unacceptable behaviour.

- Systems are in place to enable and encourage managers to deal with unacceptable behaviour.
- Systems are in place to enable and encourage employees to report unacceptable behaviour.

Roles

This is whether people understand their role within the organisation and whether the organisation ensures that the person does not have conflicting roles. Employees indicate that they understand their role and responsibilities; and systems are in place locally to respond to any individual concerns.

- The organisation ensures that, as far as possible, the different requirements it places upon employees are compatible.
- The organisation provides information to enable employees to understand their role and responsibilities.
- The organisation ensures that, as far as possible, the requirements it places upon employees are clear.
- Systems are in place to enable employees to raise concerns about any uncertainties or conflicts they have in their role and responsibilities.

Change

How organisational change (large or small) is managed and communicated in the organisation. Employees indicate that the organisation engages them frequently when undergoing an organisational change and systems are in place locally to respond to any individual concerns.

- The organisation provides employees with timely information to enable them to understand the reasons for proposed changes.
- The organisation ensures adequate employee consultation on changes and provides opportunities for employees to influence proposals.
- Employees are aware of the probable impact of any changes to their jobs. If necessary, employees are given training to support any changes in their jobs.
- Employees are aware of timetables for changes.
- Employees have access to relevant support during changes.

The Management Standards

The *Management Standards* represent a set of conditions that, if present, reflect a high level of health wellbeing and organisational performance. They:

- Demonstrate good practice through a step-by-step risk assessment approach.
- Allow assessment of the current situation using surveys and other techniques.
- Promote active discussion and work in partnership with employees to help decide on practical improvements that can be made.
- Help simplify risk assessment for work-related stress by identifying the main risk factors for work-related stress, helping employers focus on the underlying causes and their prevention and providing a

yardstick by which organisations can gauge their performance in tackling the key causes of stress.

In my view, it is one of the best Government initiatives ever to have been implemented and, if more organisations operated to these standards, a great deal of stress would be reduced and the risk of serious illness mitigated.

I remember a few years ago working for an organisation that put a great deal of pressure on their staff to perform. Little was put in place to protect the wellbeing of the people, and illness and absenteeism went through the roof. We were not allowed to use the term *stress* because apparently this was *self-induced* and, to a degree, that can be the case. However this, of course, is not *always* the case and, as described before, there are many different things that can trigger stress.

If organisations take a more responsible approach by operating to the *HSE Management Standards* and individuals take a more proactive and responsible approach to personal stress management, then the union of the two intentions could well improve the current rate of stress-related illness and absenteeism which is clearly choking the economy.

Stress Triggers

Many factors can trigger stress according to the National Health Service. These are some of the key triggers:

- Work issues.
- Money matters.
- Relationships.
- Family problems.
- Moving house.
- Bereavement.

Stress Symptoms

Stress affects different people in different ways, and everyone has a different method of dealing with it. The chemicals that are released by your body as a result of stress can build up over time and cause various mental and physical symptoms. These are listed below.

Mental Symptoms

- Anger.
- Depression.
- Anxiety.
- Changes in behaviour.
- Food cravings.
- Lack of appetite.
- Frequent crying.
- Difficulty sleeping.
- Feeling tired.
- Difficulty concentrating.

Physical Symptoms

- Chest pains.
- Constipation or diarrhoea.
- Cramps or muscle spasms.

- Dizziness.
- Fainting spells.
- Nail biting.
- Nervous twitches.
- Pins and needles.
- Feeling restless.
- A tendency to sweat.
- Sexual difficulties such as erectile dysfunction or a loss of sexual desire.
- Breathlessness.
- Muscular aches.
- Difficulty sleeping.

If you have been experiencing some of these symptoms for a long period of time you are at risk of developing high blood pressure which can lead to heart attacks and stroke.

Experiencing even one or two of these symptoms can make you feel frustrated or anxious. This can be a vicious circle - for example, you want to avoid stress but symptoms such as frequent crying or nervous twitching can make you feel annoyed with yourself and even more stressed.

Stress and Depression

Depression is a very wide topic and I don't imagine for one moment that I would be able to do it justice in this book other than to really highlight the very concerning statistics that are emerging and how mental illness is becoming more and more of an issue in the workplace.

As someone who is challenged by the illness, I have absolutely every empathy with people who experience episodes and the feeling that you are indeed the invisible patient. The fact that you can't see it is possibly one of the most frustrating aspects and makes it also very difficult for people around you, who don't get it, to understand.

Health professionals use the terms depression, depressive illness or clinical depression to refer to something very different from the common experience of feeling miserable or fed-up for a short period of time.

Some people who do not experience it themselves can be quite insensitive and intolerant and misinterpret it as weakness of character, a negative attitude or hyper-sensitivity.

There is, however, an increasing awareness of the illness and, despite the fact that it is still dogged with negative connotations, it seems that more and more people are having the courage to be more open about it which can only help other people.

Depression is quite a common condition and about 15% of people will have a bout of severe depression at some point in their lives. However, the exact number of people with depression is hard to estimate because many people do not get help, or are not formally diagnosed with the condition.

Women are twice as likely to suffer from depression

as men, although men are far more likely to commit suicide. This may be because men are more reluctant to seek help for depression.

Depression can affect people of any age, including children. Studies have shown that 2% of teenagers in the UK are affected by depression with an increasing suicide rate.

People with a family history of depression are more likely to experience depression themselves. However it is now acknowledged that high exposure to stress can trigger chemical imbalance in the brain and trigger depression. It affects people in many different ways and can cause a wide variety of physical, psychological and social symptoms.

You don't have to be a celebrity to be *bipolar* which is a form of manic depression – a condition that Stephen Fry has raised awareness of in recent years. Depression comes in different forms, affecting people in different ways and is a very real illness with consequences.It is certainly *not* a sign of failure. Winston Churchill, Abraham Lincoln, Mahatma Gandhi and Florence Nightingale all experienced bouts of depression.

It is learning to handle depression that is the key and, having experienced a particularly bad episode last year, I embarked on a voyage of discovery in terms of taking a proactive approach. Here are some personal tips from my own first-hand experience that have worked amazingly well for me and I hope will work for you too.

NB: it is also very important that you seek professional advice if you believe that you are suffering with the illness, as you may well need to be prescribed medication. However, in many cases, medication in isolation may not be enough so here are some additional strategies that you can put in place.

How to Manage Depression

✓ Wake up with an attitude of gratitude; focus on all the positive aspects in your life.
✓ Get up half an hour earlier than you would and go for a brisk walk – this works wonders!
✓ Use positive self-talk and affirmations.
✓ Avoid negative unsupportive people.
✓ Investigate any kind of CBT (Cognitive Behavioural Therapy).
✓ Avoid any counselling that is regressive.
✓ Set personal goals and focus on positive outcomes.
✓ Use positive visualisation techniques.
✓ Eliminate alcohol – it is not a good combination with depression.
✓ Drink loads of water.
✓ Manage blood-sugar levels by eating a low GI diet.
✓ Cut out refined sugar – one of the best things that you can do.
✓ Be open with people when you are depressed, but focus on getting better rather than wallowing.
✓ Take action - doing is far better than festering.
✓ Exercise – As good as a mild anti-depressant.
✓ Take a Vitamin B Complex – great for the nervous system.

✓ Hugging – physical affection is great for promoting serotonin.
✓ Keep a thought diary – write down any negative thought then play a game of how you can turn it into a positive.
✓ Remember – you are not alone.
✓ Explore the websites at the end of this book to seek further help and advice.

How to Prevent Stress

First of all, let's take a proactive approach to stress and see how it can be prevented. You may find some of the methods that are outlined below useful.

✓ Positive Self Talk

We have already established that, if the subconscious brain is told something by the conscious brain, we cannot distinguish between the actual or synthetic reality. Therefore, if you tell yourself that you are stressed, then you will be.

I have certainly worked in environments where stress is almost fashionable where everyone rushed around like a headless chicken spending more time telling everyone how stressed they were than actually doing the supposed things that are stressing them out.

That kind of culture can almost breed an epidemic of stress because everyone else then thinks that they should be stressed too. Actually working smarter, not harder, is by far the best way to prevent stress and also to listen to yourself and recognise the difference between personal pressure and real stress. So what are you telling yourself?

✓ Other People

It's amazing how *other people* can make us feel stressed either because of the way that they behave or the audience that we create in our minds that sits in judgement of our every action. Very often we will have a perception of what we believe people expect from us and, in some cases, we can be completely wrong.

There is a danger that we can put a self-imposed pressure upon ourselves because we are so concerned about what people think of us. This is where self-esteem so important and hopefully the tips in Chapter 3 will have been useful in helping you to develop your self-confidence. By balancing your personal referencing, you will find that on occasions this can take away some of the *internal pressure* that we put ourselves under.

✓ Take Responsibility

It is very easy to blame anything and everything around you for any stress you may feel. In fact, it has become such a good excuse that it can easily stop you from taking responsibility in seeking a different approach to your work that may well create a whole new work ethos for you. Whenever you feel stress, challenge the way that *you* approach the way you go about things.

As Gandhi so eloquently put it: *"Be the change you want the World to be"*.

✓ Embrace Change

One of the things that can really stress people out is change. We can become creatures of habit and we like things to remain the same, as change requires some greater effort initially. However, in an ever-evolving world, change is inevitable and keeping an open and positive mind and focussing on the positive benefits that those changes can bring can only help us to seek out opportunities and personal growth.

✓ Learn to Negotiate

One of the biggest issues that we have sometimes, especially when we want to be perceived as positive and hardworking, is to say no when we have too much on our plates. However, we have to be realistic for our own sanity. It may be that you are able to do part of something but not all of it. So - before you jump in with a definite yes or no – assess the situation and negotiate a positive win - win outcome for all concerned.

✓ Assertive Communication

Assertiveness is a great skill to have, especially when we simply do not have enough time on our hands and we have to say no to a request. Also, if you are a passive or aggressive communicator (as you will have found out in Chapter 3) poor communication skills can add to your stress levels.

✓ Deep Breathing

If you feel yourself getting stressed, try to halt those feelings in their tracks by relaxing your muscles and taking deep breaths. Start by inhaling for three seconds, then exhale for a little longer. This will help to remove the older oxygen from your lungs and replace it with fresh oxygen that will improve your circulation and alertness. Continue these deep breathing exercises until you feel calmer and ready to continue what you were doing. It might be better to do something else rather than continue with the stressful task.

✓ Healthy Eating

It is so important to eat a healthy, balanced diet when you are stressed because food and drink can have a big impact on the way that you feel and act. Some people find that stress causes them to snack on sugary, unhealthy foods such as crisps and biscuits. This gives your body a sugar rush followed by a sharp drop in your sugar and energy levels. However, this can make you feel tired or irritable, as well as making it harder for you to concentrate.

Eating at regular times and not skipping meals can make a big difference. This will allow your body to release a steady stream of energy throughout the day which will help improve your concentration and mood.

It's widely accepted that nutritional deficiency impairs the health of the body, and it's unrealistic not to expect the brain to be affected as well by poor diet. If the brain is affected, so are our thoughts, feelings and behaviour.

We know that certain vitamins and minerals are

required to ensure healthy brain and neurological functionality. We know also that certain deficiencies relate directly to specific brain and nervous system weaknesses: The Vitamin B Group is particularly relevant to the brain, depression and stress susceptibility. Vitamin B1 deficiency is associated with depression, nervous system weakness and dementia. B2 deficiency is associated with nervous system disorders and depression.

B3 is essential for protein synthesis, including the neurotransmitter serotonin, which is necessary for maintaining a healthy nervous system. Vitamin B6 is essential for neurotransmitter synthesis and maintaining a healthy nervous system; B6 deficiency is associated with depression and dementia. B12 deficiency is associated with peripheral nerve degeneration, dementia, and depression.

Vitamin C is essential to protect against stress too: it maintains a healthy immune system, which is important for reducing stress susceptibility (we are more likely to suffer from stress when we are ill, and we are more prone to illness when our immune system is weak). Vitamin C speeds healing which contributes to reducing stress susceptibility. Vitamin C is associated with improving post-traumatic stress disorders and chronic infections.

A 2003 UK 18 month study into violent and anti-social behaviour at a youth offenders' institution provided remarkable evidence as to the link between diet and stress: Around 230 inmate volunteers were divided into two groups. Half were given a daily vitamin/fatty acid/mineral supplement; half were given a placebo. The group given the supplement showed a 25% reduction in recorded offences, and a 40% reduction in serious cases including violence towards others, behaviours that are directly attributable to stress.

Vitamin D helps maintain healthy body condition, particularly bones and speed of fracture healing, which are directly linked to stress susceptibility.

An adequate intake of minerals is also essential for a healthy body and brain, and so for reducing stress susceptibility.

A proper balanced diet is clearly essential, both to avoid direct physical stress causes via brain and nervous system, and to reduce stress susceptibility resulting from poor health and condition. Processed foods are not as good for you as fresh natural foods. Look at all the chemicals listed on the packaging to see what you are putting into your body.

The rule is simple and inescapable: eat and drink healthily, and avoid excessive intake of toxins, to reduce stress susceptibility and stress itself. If you are suffering from stress and not obeying this simple rule, you will continue to be stressed and, moreover, you will maintain a higher susceptibility to stress.

Irrespective of your tastes, it's easy these days to have a balanced healthy diet if you want to - the challenge isn't in knowing what's good and bad, it's simply a matter of commitment and personal resolve. You have one body for the whole of your life - look after it.

✓ Reduce Caffeine

Caffeine can exacerbate or even cause stress, anxiety, depression and insomnia because it interferes with a tranquilising neurotransmitter chemical in the brain called adenosine. This is the chemical which turns down our anxiety levels - it's our body's version of a tranquiliser. Caffeine docks into a receptor for adenosine and regular use of caffeine is enough to produce anxiety and depression in susceptible individuals.

Research has indicated that caffeine increases the secretion of stress hormones like adrenaline, so if you are already secreting higher stress hormones, caffeine will boost it even higher and exacerbate stress/anxiety or depression even further than it already is. By eventually cutting caffeine you will lower your stress hormone levels and therefore reduce stress, anxiety and depression.

✓ Reduce Alcohol

Alcohol, when consumed in large amounts, stimulates the hypothalamus, adrenal and pituitary glands and one result of this is an increased level of both cortisol and adrenaline within the body. But both play a significant role in reinforcing the symptoms of stress.

✓ Exercise

The benefits of exercise are numerous, as I hope I have already expressed. Not only does it release a chemical called serotonin, which makes you feel happier and less stressed, it also improves circulation and prevents conditions such as stroke and heart attack. Exercise also allows you to take out your frustration and anger in a constructive way through a very positive channel.

In particular, fast walking has been found to be very beneficial for relieving stress, as well as being an effective method of weight control.

✓ Sleep

It is common for your sleep pattern to be disturbed when you are feeling stressed. If you are worried about something, it can often be on your mind even when you try to forget about it. This may cause sleepless nights or bad dreams. You may find it difficult getting to sleep or you may wake up a few times during the night. This can also make you tired and groggy the next day, which can make you feel even more stressed. In fact sleep deprivation can *cause* stress – here are a few tips to help you.

How to Sleep Better

✓ Go to bed and get up at about the same time every day, even on the weekends. Sticking to a schedule helps reinforce your body's sleep-wake cycle and can help you fall asleep better at night.

✓ Don't eat or drink large amounts before bedtime. Eat a light dinner about two hours before sleeping. If you're prone to heartburn, avoid spicy or fatty foods, which can make your heartburn flare and prevent a restful sleep. Also, limit how much you drink before bed. Too much liquid can cause you to wake up repeatedly during the night for trips to the bathroom.

✓ Avoid nicotine, caffeine and alcohol in the evening. These are stimulants that can keep you awake. Smokers often experience withdrawal symptoms at night, and smoking in bed is dangerous. Avoid caffeine for eight hours before your planned bedtime. Your body doesn't store caffeine, but it takes many hours to eliminate the stimulant and its effects. And, although often believed to be a sedative, alcohol actually disrupts sleep.

✓ Exercise regularly. Regular physical activity, especially aerobic exercise, can help you fall asleep faster and make your sleep more restful. Don't exercise within three hours of your bedtime, however. Exercising right before bed may make getting to sleep more difficult.

✓ Make your bedroom cool, dark, quiet and comfortable. Create a room that's ideal for sleeping. Adjust the lighting, temperature, humidity and noise level to your preferences. Use blackout curtains, eye covers, earplugs, extra blankets, a fan, a humidifier or other devices to create an environment that suits your needs.

✓ Sleep primarily at night. Daytime naps may steal hours from night-time slumber. Limit daytime sleep to about a half-hour and make it during mid-afternoon. If you work nights, keep your window coverings closed so that sunlight, which adjusts the body's internal clock, doesn't interrupt your sleep. If you have a day job and sleep at night, but still have trouble waking up, leave the window coverings open and let the sunlight help wake you up.

✓ Choose a comfortable mattress and pillow. Features of a good bed are subjective and differ for each person. But make sure you have a bed that's comfortable. If you share your bed, make sure there's enough room for two. Children and pets are often disruptive, so you may need to set limits on how often they sleep in bed with you.

✓ Start a relaxing bedtime routine. Do the same things each night to tell your body it's time to wind down. This may include taking a warm bath or shower, reading a book, or listening to soothing music. Relaxing activities done with lowered lights can help ease the transition between wakefulness and sleepiness.

✓ Go to bed when you're tired and turn out the lights. If you don't fall asleep within 15 to 20 minutes, get up and do something else. Go back to bed when you're tired. Don't agonise over falling asleep. The stress will only prevent sleep.

✓ Use sleeping pills only as a last resort. Check with your doctor before taking any sleep medications.

✓ **Quit Smoking**

Contrary to popular belief, smoking does not help to combat stress. In fact, it can make stress worse and it causes damage to your body. Giving up smoking is not easy and, in the short term, may lead to you feeling more stressed, or annoyed. However, you should remember that the irritability and craving is a sign that your body is trying to repair itself.

If you would like more information, or advice, about quitting smoking, you can call the NHS Stop Smoking Helpline on 0800 0224 332.

✓ Relaxation

When you are stressed, your muscles often tense, which can cause muscular aches to develop later on. When you feel yourself getting stressed, shrug your shoulders a few times and shake out your arms and legs. This will help to loosen your muscles.

Some people find that it helps them to relax if they imagine a peaceful place, such as a desert island or a tranquil lake. Imagine yourself being there and the scenery around you. Diverting your mind to a calming environment will help to distract you from the stress and relax your body.

✓ Humour

Humour is one of the greatest and quickest devices for reducing stress. It works because laughter produces helpful chemicals in the brain. Humour also gets your brain thinking and working in a different way - it distracts you from having a stressed mindset. Distraction is a simple effective de-stressor - it takes your thoughts away from the stress, and thereby diffuses the stressful feelings.

Therefore, most people will feel quite different and notice a change in mindset after laughing and being distracted by something humorous.

✓ Drink Water!

Remember Dr Batman - *Your body's many cries for water*. Go get a big cup or a bottle of water now. Most of us fail to drink enough water - that's water - not tea, coffee or fruit juice. All of your organs, including your brain, are strongly dependent on water to function properly. It's how we are built. If you starve your body of water you will function below your best - and you will get stressed, physically and mentally.

Offices and workplaces commonly have a very dry atmosphere due to air-conditioning, etc., which increases people's susceptibility to de-hydration. This is why you must keep your body properly hydrated by regularly drinking water (most people need 8 glasses of water a day).

You will drink more water if you keep some on your desk at all times – it's human nature to drink it if it's there - so go get some *now*. When you drink water, you need to eliminate, so this gives you a bit of a break and a bit of exercise now and then, which also reduces stress.

When you pee you can see if your body is properly hydrated (your pee will be clear or near clear - if it's yellow, you are not taking enough water). You do not need to buy expensive mineral water. Tap water is fine.

✓ **Crying**
I call this the detoxification of the soul. When you are feeling really tense or stressed, a good cry can work wonders. This is easier for women than men. Not much is known about the physiology of crying and tears, although many find that crying - weeping proper tears - has a powerful, helpful effect on stress levels. Whatever the science behind crying, a good

bout of sobbing and weeping does seem to release tension for many people.

Of course how and where you choose to submit to this most basic of emotional impulses is up to you. The middle of the boardroom during an important presentation to a top client is probably not a great idea!

It is a shame that attitudes towards crying and tears prevent many people from crying, and it's a sad reflection on our unforgiving society that some people who might benefit from a good cry feel that they shouldn't do it ever - even in complete privacy. Unfortunately, most of us - especially boys - are told as children that crying is bad or shameful or childish, which of course is utter nonsense. Arguably only the bravest cry unashamedly - the rest of us would rather suffer than appear weak, which is daft, but nevertheless real.

Whatever, shedding a few tears can be a very good thing now and then, and if you've yet to discover its benefits then give it a try. You might be surprised.

✓ Anger Management
The term *anger management* is widely used now as if the subject stands alone. Celebrities with volatile temperaments have hit the news and it is clearly something that affects people in the workplace especially when it manifests itself because of stress.

However, "anger management" is simply an aspect of managing stress, since anger in the workplace is a symptom of stress.

Anger is often stress in denial, and as such is best approached via one-to-one counselling. Training courses can convey anger management and stress reduction theory and ideas, but one-to-one counselling is necessary to turn theory into practice. Management of anger (and any other unreasonable emotional behaviour for that matter) and the stress that causes it, can only be improved if the person wants to change by acceptance, cognisance and commitment. Awareness is the first requirement.

Some angry people take pride in their anger and don't want to change; others fail to appreciate the effect on self and others. Without a commitment to change, there's not a lot that a manager or employer can do to help; anger management is only possible when the angry person accepts and commits to the need to change.

A big factor in persuading someone of the need to commit to change is to look objectively and sensitively with the other person at the consequences (for themselves and others) of their anger. Often angry people are in denial ("my temper is okay") and put it down to acceptable mood swings, so removing this denial is essential. Helping angry people to realise that their behaviour is destructive and negative is an important first step. Discuss the effects on their health and their co-workers. Get the person to see things from outside themselves.

As with stress, the next anger management step is for the angry person to understand the cause of their angry tendency, which will be a combination of stressors and stress susceptibility factors. Angry people need help in gaining this understanding - the counsellor often won't know the reason either until rapport is established.

If the problem is a temporary tendency then short-term acute stress may be the direct cause. Use one-to-one counselling to discover the causes and then agree necessary action to deal with them. Where the anger is persistent, frequent and ongoing, long-term chronic stress is more likely to be the cause. Again, counselling is required to get to the root causes. Exposing these issues can be very difficult, so great sensitivity is required. The counsellor may need several sessions in order to build sufficient trust and rapport.

The situation must be referred to a suitably qualified person whenever necessary, i.e. when the counsellor is unable to establish a rapport, analyse the causes, or agree a way forward. In any event, if you spot the need for anger management in a person, be aware that serious anger, and especially violence, is a clinical problem and so must be referred to a suitably qualified advisor or support group - under no circumstances attempt to deal with seriously or violently angry people via workplace counselling; these cases require expert professional help.

Establishing commitment to change and identifying the causes is sufficient for many people to make changes and improve - the will to change, combined with awareness of causes, then leads to a solution.

✓ Time Management

One of the biggest challenges that many people face is personal time management and the ability to prioritise. Let's face it; we all have our own quirky little habits that we have adopted and I am sure we have all been guilty of putting ourselves and other people under unnecessary pressure by just not being as well-organised as we could.

Here are few tips that may help:

Planning

- ✓ Identify the individual tasks that will ensure you achieve your goal. Put them in a logical order (identify those which have to be completed before the next can be started and those that can be done in parallel).
- ✓ Identify the critical path – the sequence of events that dictates the fastest time in which an entire plan can be completed. Work backwards from the last task to the beginning of your plan.
- ✓ Add estimates of resources – (costs, people, and time) and be realistic.

✓ Put your tasks on a timeline and estimate completion date.

✓ Check that the resources are sufficient to run the plan – if not can you delay some non critical tasks to smooth the resource demands.

✓ Identify risks in your plan and build in contingencies.

✓ Make it clear which tasks are contingencies – you can remove them later to gain more confidence in your plan.

✓ Identify who needs to know what to make your plan successful – how are you going to keep them up to date.

✓ Keep your eye fixed on the overall goal and add shortcuts along the way – be flexible.

✓ Make your plan enjoyable so it is more likely to succeed.

✓ Design your plans so that they can be changed easily if necessary.

✓ Review your plans on a regular basis to check your progress.

✓ Monitor what really happens as you go along. It will show you if your planning is accurate or needs amending to fit reality.

✓ Make sure the level of detail in your plan is useful.

✓ Use other people – delegate to people that can do a specific job better than you.

Prioritisation

✓ Make a list of your current projects and make some time every week to review progress.

✓ Check your strategies for identifying the highest priority tasks.

✓ Develop a clear set of criteria by asking yourself 'what is important to me about this?'

Pareto Analysis

✓ Make sure your maximum effort is focused on the area that will give you the biggest return. Pareto was an Italian tax collector in the middle ages. He discovered that 80% of the money he collected came from 20% of his richest clients. By focusing on these he was able to use his time most effectively.

✓ Use Pareto analysis as one of your criteria to help you prioritise.

✓ Work out what takes up most of your time and tackle it first. A 10% improvement in something which takes you 10 weeks will save you a whole week!

✓ When deciding between several tasks ask 'which will help me achieve my goal?'

Contingency

✓ Check your estimating – estimate how long something will take e.g. a phone call and then record how long it actually took.

✓ Improve your estimating by checking your estimates and adjusting them accordingly next time. This will improve your planning skills.

✓ Identify your critical tasks and likely trouble spots in your plan before you start.

✓ Design monitoring systems to alert you before a problem arises so you can take action.
✓ Have contingency plans ready to help you achieve your goals.

Motivating Yourself

✓ Focus on how great it will be once it is done not how much you hate doing it.
✓ Break tasks up you do not like up into very small packages and do them on a daily basis.

Concentration

✓ How long is your attention span? Start working on a task, make note of the time you start, when your mind starts to wander take note of the time. Do this for a few tasks to find your attention span.
✓ Plan all of your tasks to fit with your attention span. Break larger tasks into smaller chunks to fit in with your attention span.
✓ Do something physical to keep you motivated – after each task, do something physical (even filing) but a walk is ideal.
✓ Is there a time when you work better e.g. first thing in the morning? If you are struggling with something in the late afternoon, leave it to the evening and complete a less demanding task.
✓ Make sure you drink enough water – 2 litres a day to boost concentration.

Your Diary

✓ Make sure you keep it up to date.

✓ As soon as you agree to do something, put it in your diary.
✓ Put reminders into your diary – such as insurance renewals and events you are likely to forget.

Filing

✓ Put the files you use most often near to you, the ones you hardly use can be stored in a separate room or can be archived.
✓ When it takes too long to find a document, reorganise that file into smaller files.
✓ Create a file for regular meetings. This will save you time when preparing for the meeting.
✓ Work out what you really need in a filing system – e.g. do you really need to be able to retrieve info while you are on the phone?
✓ Analyse what is causing you the biggest problem and concentrate on that first.
✓ Work out a regime to get rid of that huge pile and work on it a little every day.

Email

✓ Unsubscribe from mail outs and newsletters that do not interest you.
✓ Decrease the volume of emails you send by only replying if you need to comment, do not reply to all unless necessary.
✓ Use flags to highlight emails that are a priority.
✓ Do not pass on an email just to get it out of your inbox.

Interruptions

✓ Work out who interrupts you the most and why – what can you do to prevent it?

✓ If people ask you for the same info all the time could you produce it in written form? Or is it that you don't explain it properly? Could they get it elsewhere?

✓ Let people know when it is convenient to be interrupted and when it is not.

✓ Plan regular fixed meetings with the people who interrupt you frequently so they can save their questions instead.

✓ Check your body language – do you sit when someone interrupts you? This gives them the power – stand and walk towards them instead.

✓ Get back to people when you say you will. This reduces people interrupting you.

✓ Do you tend to offer people help before they ask? This may make them dependent on you and give you extra work.

✓ When someone interrupts you say "I have two minutes, if it will take longer, lets arrange a time". Get your diary out.

✓ Are you a control freak? – not all decisions have to be made by you – delegate!

✓ Turn off your email alarm and check emails several times a day rather than every time they arise.

✓ Use your voice mail to avoid being interrupted.

✓ If you have trouble saying no, then negotiate. Ask people what needs to be achieved.

Managing your Manager

✓ Never wait for your manager to come to you to complain about something – always tell your manager about problems yourself.

✓ Always imagine things from your manager's perspective.

✓ Keep your manager appraised of your plans and where you are on them.

✓ Let your manager know in advance if you are going to slip timescales.

✓ Ask your manager how they would like to be kept informed of your progress.

✓ Ask your manager what you could do to improve your service to them – then do it!

✓ Find out what is important to your manager – once you know focus on that aspect of your work.

Meetings

✓ Make sure there is an agenda and send it to people in advance.

✓ Allot time to each agenda item.

✓ Make your objectives clear.

✓ Give people an idea of how long you expect their contributions to be and time them.

✓ Make sure you give everyone a chance to speak to reduce interruptions.

✓ Monitor the time carefully – if it starts to overrun explain the fact and ask people to be brief. If necessary reschedule some items.

✓ Get all actions and agreements minuted and read each out at the end of that agenda point.

✓ Send out the minutes within a few days of the meeting.

Reading

✓ Be clear about your objective for reading a document before you start.
✓ Read the abstract and conclusion with your objective in mind – throw it away if nothing there helps you.
✓ Skim large documents as often the important info will be in one part.
✓ Keep documents you want to refer to later in one file
✓ If you travel with work often, use this time to read.
✓ Throw away anything you can and plan the reading you need to do.
✓ Work out how long your reading will take.
✓ With all reading tasks do it just once. E.g. when you get an email don't read it then put it away and come back to it. You will only have to read it again.

Set Goals

Setting personal goals and tracking them effectively and efficiently means that you can manage your time more effectively and keep focused on what is important.

Give your stress wings and let it fly away.
—Carin Hartness

How to Work Wonders
with Stress

- ✓ Understand your stress trigger.
- ✓ Take proactive steps to address stress before it happens.
- ✓ Use breathing techniques.
- ✓ Learn to use relaxation techniques.
- ✓ Reduce caffeine.
- ✓ Reduce alcohol.
- ✓ Quit smoking.
- ✓ Eat a well balanced diet.
- ✓ Manage blood sugar levels.
- ✓ Eat a good breakfast.
- ✓ Sleep 6-8 hours a day.
- ✓ Drink camomile tea.
- ✓ Keep well-hydrated.
- ✓ Use positive self-talk to manage stress.
- ✓ Time-manage effectively.
- ✓ Learn to negotiate.
- ✓ Exercise and keep active.
- ✓ Don't spread your stress.
- ✓ Maintain a positive attitude.

CHAPTER FIVE - ENVIRONMENT

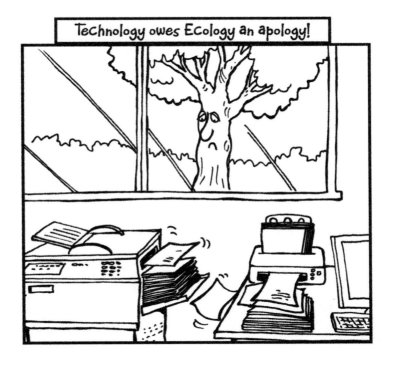

Modern technology owes ecology an apology

Alan M Eddison

It makes sense that people who are happy within their working environment will work far more effectively and happily than those who are uncomfortable. As I have outlined in Chapter 4, your work environment can also have a big impact on your stress levels.

Creating an environment that is comfortable and stimulating and conducive to both physical and psychological wellbeing is so important. This will contribute significantly to that all important 'feel good factor' at work.

I am sure that we have all worked in different work environments and some will certainly be better than others. Having worked with a real cross-section of organisations, I have seen some really impressive examples of environments where you can literally feel the positive effect that it has on their staff and actually reflects upon staff morale and retention.

Also taking into consideration the environment and the impact that we have on it is very important these days if we are to protect the world that we live in.

So taking a really good look at your work environment and what you can do to make improvements or offer suggestions to your organisation is a great contribution.

Wastage is a huge issue in western society and I came across a rather sad statistic that stated that, apparently, a third of the food that we buy in the UK ends up being thrown away – and sadder still is the fact that most of it could have been eaten. Looking after the environment isn't about turning yourself in an eco warrior – it is more about doing your bit to contribute to the sustainability of human survival.

You have possibly already taken steps to reduce the amount of energy you use at home, but what can you do at work? It's equally important to make a difference there and, if you're not in a position to make the changes that will cut your company's carbon footprint, then try to raise awareness and encourage your organisation to take more responsibility for the environment.

Here are some ideas for a cleaner, greener, more climate-friendly workplace. If we all do our bit it can make a huge difference.

How to be Environmentally Friendly

✓ Switch off Lights and Equipment
How many office buildings and shops do you see all lit up long after the employees have gone home?

Lighting an average-sized empty office overnight wastes enough electricity to make 1,000 hot drinks or print 800 sheets of paper. One solution is to appoint someone (on a rota) to ensure everything is turned off at the end of the day and during the day if it's not needed. If you have cleaners who come in after hours, ensure they do the same. Occupancy sensors work well for some businesses (the lights only come on in rooms or areas in use) and, if your workplace has lots of windows, do you even need the lights on at all, especially in summer?

Putting your computer into sleep mode will reduce the amount of energy it uses by 60-70 per cent. And, if you can, turn it off. After just 16 minutes of not using your computer, it's more energy efficient to turn it off and restart it than to keep it on. Most IT equipment now has power-management features, so make sure these are activated on yours.

✓ Unplug Chargers
You may not realise it but laptop and mobile phone chargers continue to charge (using up to 95 per cent of the power) even when no longer attached to the device. So you must remember to unplug chargers and, if you turn your mobile phones and BlackBerries off at night, you'll only have to charge them half as much.

✓ Print Responsibly
Printing emails is often unnecessary and a waste of both paper and electricity. How many times have you printed a whole chain of emails, spanning many

pages, when you only wanted the first one or two? Think before you print and, whatever the document is, consider whether you need a hard copy or can manage without.

If you do have to print emails, ensure you only print the pages you need, or paste the relevant sections into a Word document and only print that. Find out if your office has duplex printers, which print double sided. They halve paper use and reduce energy consumption by an estimated 25 per cent.

✓ Recycle in the Office

The UK has one of the worst recycling records in Europe, so more businesses recycling would make a dramatic difference. Providing recycling bins for paper is an obvious and essential measure (the average Briton uses more than 200kg of paper each year and yet only around 65 per cent of this is recycled), but businesses can have a much bigger impact.

UK businesses throw away more than 1.5 million computers every year. More than 90 per cent of these are fully functioning and less than 5 per cent are refurbished for reuse. And don't forget that office essentials such as printer cartridges can also be refilled and reused.

Set up recycling bins for glass, cans, plastic, cardboard, etc in your office.

✓ Think before you Travel

Is your business trip really necessary? Or is there an

equally effective way you can communicate? Lots of business is traditionally done face to face but, in this technological age, need it be? The usual modes of business travel, car and plane, won't help you reduce your company's carbon footprint.

Flying from Glasgow to London, for example, generates six times as much carbon dioxide as going by train. Taking the train also saves you time, as there are no lengthy check-in queues or security checks, and you can work more easily on the train, so travelling time is more productive. And let's not forget that flying business class is one of the most carbon-intensive ways to travel.

Aim to reduce your CO_2 emissions from business travel by managing the absolute need to travel and by providing alternative means of communication, such as video conferencing. If you don't have video conferencing facilities in your office, suites can be hired for a nominal rate as opposed to £150 an hour. It's the next best thing to face-to-face meetings and the benefits are not just environmental but economic too. For larger corporations in particular, installing unlimited video-conferencing facilities can result in major savings in annual travel costs, as well as reduced CO_2 emissions.

The CO_2 emissions produced from travelling to and from work are equally important to address. Organise car-sharing, cycle, walk or use public transport. The savings made can be up to 0.5kg of CO_2 for every mile you don't drive. Employers can help too, by providing loans for season railcards and gradually reducing spaces for parking.

✓ Wrap Up
Rather than ramping up the heating in the office (which isn't great for your health) wear layers to work. Better still, encourage your work colleagues to go on a walk around the block in the morning with you to warm up before work so that your body temperature is naturally higher.

✓ Buy Green Electricity
Have you thought about getting your company to switch to green electricity? Most energy suppliers offer competitive tariffs that provide green or renewable energy to help considerably reduce your carbon footprint. Energy generated from the sun, wind or water produces fewer or no CO_2 emissions. By purchasing electricity from these renewable sources, your organisation would be helping to increase the global investment in and supply of renewable energy.

✓ Champion Change
We can all play a part in reducing our carbon footprint at work. From buying green electricity to switching your computer off at night, every little helps. Raising awareness through events is a great way of getting others in your organisation to play their part and champion change. Why not take part in World Environment Day, the United Nations Environment Programme's international environmental awareness-raising day. This takes place on the 5th June every year.

✓ Share Ideas

There are so many great initiatives that organisations are doing to support the environment and sharing ideas *is* a great idea. There will be lots of people within your organisation that may well have some great suggestions. Try to encourage your organisation to get people together to share best practice and to generally raise awareness and encourage environmental responsibility. The best companies to work for are organisations who take responsibility and many people these days take this into consideration when selecting a company to work for.

How to Make Your Workplace Physically Better

✓ Noise

If you feel that you may have a problem with the amount of noise within your workplace then you need to get a measurement of noise levels done by a competent person. Noise can be the cause of irreversible hearing damage and also lead to increased levels of stress. Noise is normally caused by loud machines so, when buying any new plant or machinery, remember to check the noise emission levels. The remedies are usually quite simple e.g. providing your employees with hearing protection, rotating the staff who work close to noisy machinery to decrease their exposure times, and clearly marking any "high noise" areas to warn people of the risk.

✓ Ventilation

Fresh air is one of the most important elements of a working environment for several reasons:

- Respiration.
- The removal of excess heat.
- The dilution of various airborne impurities (dust, fumes, tobacco smoke, body odour).

Adequate ventilation can be provided by simply allowing windows to be opened. Air conditioning systems cannot be counted as fresh air systems as the air is recirculated and therefore not as effective, particularly as it can still carry germs and other impurities.

✓ Temperature
The minimum temperature for sedentary work is 16 Celsius (about 60 degrees Fahrenheit) and, for work involving physical effort, the minimum should be 13 Celsius (about 55 degrees Fahrenheit). Thermometers should be provided to allow monitoring of these levels.

✓ Tidiness
Take responsibility to keep your work area tidy. Always put things back where you found them. Clear up if you make a drink and be as under tidiness as possible. You will feel so much better and it is also much more considerate to those around you.

✓ Pictures
Visual images at work can really work well in raising morale. Positive pictures with happy faces and beautiful scenery can help to promote a good atmosphere. In some organisations, posters with motivational quotes are hung up to inspire people and to reinforce a positive mental attitude – I have

also seen the poem *Desiderata* framed and put up in many offices – this is a wonderful and inspirational poem that you will find in the back of this book.

✓ Lighting

There are various reasons why lighting is important in the workplace which include the illumination of potential hazards, and to prevent eye strain. There are various other considerations such as the facts that fluorescent lighting should not flicker, there should be no glare, and there should be no sudden contrast in levels of lighting. All light fittings should be kept clean and ideally the ceiling should be light-coloured to reflect the light.

✓ Music

Music in a work setting can be very beneficial and can improve productivity. Studies have shown that music in the workplace promotes positive mood, sense of team, improves alertness and can lessen the event of accidents. Obviously this needs to be appropriate as, in some work environments, it would be completely unsuitable and employers do need to consider the type of music played. The mood and style should fit the business. Experts suggest all-instrumental soundtracks so that workers don't become distracted by the lyrics.

✓ Laughter

It is important to remember that your behaviour in the workplace is part of what makes the environment a good place to be. If everyone at work is happy and positive and friendly then the chances are it is going

to be a much better place to be. Laughter, for example, can be a very positive environment enhancer. Some organisations may frown upon the idea of laughter at work, seeing it as a distraction from getting the work done. The work ethic many of us were raised with also reinforces this attitude as "Work isn't supposed to be fun!"
Well why not?

I do believe we are starting to realise that all this suffering is really bad for us. Not only that, but we're finding that it's actually counter-productive to delivering the bottom-line results.

Scientific research points to a better way of living and working. A recent study conducted at financial institutions in America found that managers who facilitated the highest level of employee performance used humour the most often.

Scientific data also proves laughter to be an integral part of physical wellness. Dr. William Fry of Stanford University has demonstrated that laughing 200 times burns off the same amount of calories as ten minutes on the rowing machine.

Another study reveals that, after a bout of laughter, blood pressure drops to a lower, healthier level than before the laughter began. Laughter also oxygenates your blood (and thus increases your energy level), relaxes your muscles and works out all major internal systems like the cardiovascular and respiratory systems.

Furthermore, researchers report that laughter also affects the immune system. According to Dr. Lee Berk of the Loma Linda School of Public Health in California, laughing makes it grow stronger, with the body's T-cells, natural killer cells and antibodies all showing signs of increased activity.

As more and more groups realise the benefits of laughter, they incorporate it into their wellness programmes and day-to-day work. I've found from working with many organisations that they often have a lot of funny and resourceful people who just need to be given permission and encouragement to use their sense of humour on the job.

So why not look at introducing humour and fun into to your work environment?

How to be Happy at Work

✓ Make Friends
"Do you have a best friend at work?" Liking and enjoying your co-workers are hallmarks of a positive, happy work experience. Take time to get to know them. You might actually like and enjoy them. Your network provides support, resources, sharing and caring.

✓ Do Something You Enjoy Every Single Day
You may or may not love your current job and you may or may not believe that you can find something in your current job to love, but you can. Trust me. Take a look at yourself, your skills and interests, and

find something that you can enjoy doing every day. If you do something you enjoy every single day, your current job won't seem so bad.

✓ **Take Charge of Your Own Personal Development**
You are the person with the most to gain from continuing to develop professionally. Take charge of your own growth. Ask for specific and meaningful help from your boss, but march to the music of your personally developed plan and goals. You have the most to gain from growing - and the most to lose, if you stand still. Learning with others can also create a great team environment.

✓ **Take Responsibility for Knowing What Is Happening at Work**
Seek out the information you need to work effectively. Develop an information network and use it. Assertively request a weekly meeting with your boss and ask questions to learn. You are in charge of the information you receive.

✓ **Learn to Negotiate and Make Only Commitments You Can Keep**
One of the most serious causes of work stress and unhappiness is failing to keep commitments. Many employees spend more time making excuses for failing to keep a commitment, and worrying about the consequences of not keeping a commitment, than they do performing the tasks promised. Create a system of organisation and planning that enables you to assess your ability to complete a requested commitment. Don't volunteer if you don't have time.

If your workload is exceeding your available time and energy, make a comprehensive plan to ask the boss for help and resources. Don't wallow in the swamp of unkept promises.

✓ Choose to Be Happy at Work

Happiness is largely a choice. I can hear many of you arguing with me, but it's true. You can choose to be happy at work. I wish all of you had the best employer in the world, however you may not. Nevertheless, thinking positively about your work and dwelling on the aspects of your work you like will help hugely. Don't get embroiled in critical behaviour and whinging. We can all find a wealth of things to complain about if we look hard enough. Find co-workers you like and enjoy and spend your time with them. Your choices at work largely define your experience. You can choose to be happy at work. Work is what YOU make it.

> *We do not inherit the earth from our ancestors, we borrow it from our children.*
>
> —*Native American Proverb*

How to Work Wonders with your Environment

✓ Switch off lights and equipment.

✓ Unplug your chargers.

✓ Print responsibly.

✓ Recycle wherever possible.

✓ Think before you travel.

✓ Wrap up in the Winter.

✓ Buy green electricity.

✓ Champion environmentally-friendly practice.

✓ Share ideas of best practice.

✓ Be conscious of noise.

✓ Get lots of fresh air in the Summer.

✓ Put positive pictures up.

✓ Ensure the correct lighting.

✓ Play music if appropriate.

✓ Cultivate laughter in the workplace.

✓ Take responsibility for your behaviour.

✓ Project positive energy and radiate your environment.

CHAPTER SIX - GOAL SETTING

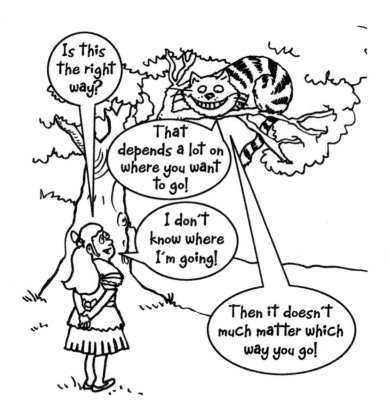

If a man knows not
what harbour he seeks,
any wind is the right wind

Seneca

At the end of each busy working day some of us may find that although we feel like we have spent the whole day working hard, we have not really accomplished as much as we think we have or would like to. Why is that? Most likely, your answer is related to goal-setting. You may work hard and keep busy, but if you do not set goals you are apt to find yourself working hard without any meaningful results or at least not establishing your point of success and job satisfaction.

Think about the story of Alice in Wonderland, when Alice first encountered the Cheshire cat in Wonderland, she asked:

"Would you tell me, please, which way I ought to go from here?"

"That depends a good deal on where you want to get to," said the Cat.

"I don't much care where," said Alice.

"Then it doesn't matter which way you go," said the Cat.

"So long as I get somewhere," Alice added as an explanation.

"Oh, you're sure to do that," said the Cat, "If you only walk long enough."

Without goals, we are like Alice – wandering aimlessly throughout life. Your brain is a goal seeking mechanism. Your ability to set goals is your master skill. Goals unlock your positive mind and release energies and ideas for success and achievement. Without goals, you simply drift and flow on the currents of life. With goals, you fly like an arrow, straight and true to your target. Setting goals gives us direction, purpose and focus in our lives.

What are the key Benefits of Setting Goals?

✓ Clarity
Setting goals requires you to develop clarity. This is the first and most important step to creating a life that you love and want.

✓ Focus
You will develop a stronger FOCUS: whatever you focus on, you get more of; if you have clear goals and focus on them, you will get more of what you DO want (your goals) and less of what you don't want.

✓ Efficiency
When you get clear about where you want to go, you set up steps and actions to get there. This increases your efficiency because you are working on what is

really important. When you work on what's important, you will accomplish more than you ever expected.

✓ Dreams
You will get what you *really* want in life, rather than settling for "whatever comes you way".

✓ Increased Self Confidence
As you set and reach goals, you become more confident in your ability to do what you say and get what you want in life. Success breeds more success.

✓ Results
Only 3% of people have proper written goals, and according to research, these people accomplish 80% more than those who don't. That's an astounding difference, isn't it?

How to Set Goals

A common acronym in goal setting is the possibly familiar **SMART goals**, but what does it really mean and what is so smart about them?

The SMART acronym is used to describe what experts consider to be "good" goal statements because they contain most of the essential ingredients. Out of all the formulas I have come across for objective and goal-seeking, it is by far the best and the most easy to apply and stick to.

The **SMART** acronym itself has several different variations depending on who you ask. However,

I think it is useful to look at all of them because it provides a well-rounded goal statement.

S Specific & significant
M Measurable, motivational, methodical & meaningful
A Action-oriented & achievable
R Realistic, relevant & recorded
T Time-bound & tangible

Writing SMART Goals

Let's take a closer look at each of these properties...

Specific - Your SMART goal statement should be a clear and specific statement of what you want.

The main reason is that your brain behaves as a goal seeking mechanism, similar to a precision guided missile. As these missiles fly, they continually make small adjustments and corrections to their trajectories to realign themselves to their target.

Your brain also works in a similar way. Dr Maxwell Maltz, author of the classic *Psycho-Cybernetics,* said that human beings have a built-in goal-seeking "success mechanism" that is part of the subconscious mind.

This success mechanism is constantly searching for ways to help us reach our targets and find answers to our problems. According to Maltz, we work and feel better when our success mechanism is fully engaged going after clear targets.

All we have to do to use this mechanism is to give it a specific target. Without one, our success mechanism lies dormant, or worse, pursues targets we didn't consciously choose.

When your target is vague or ambiguous, your success mechanism can become confused and either shut down or go after the wrong target.

Significant - Significant goals are the ones that will make a positive difference in your life. If a goal is not significant, why are you even contemplating it? Is it really your goal?

Measurable - There is an old saying that says "What gets measured gets done".

Making your goal measurable helps you **see your progress**, recognise if you are moving in the right direction, and see how far you still need to go. Some types of goals, like saving a certain amount of money each month, or reading 100 pages per week, are very easy to measure, while other goals aren't really measurable directly.

For example, if your goal is to improve your relationship with your one of your colleagues, how do you measure it?

One option is to use some sort of rating. For example, you could say that your relationship is a 6 and your goal is to make it an 8. The problem is that these types of ratings are very subjective, can change from day to day, and don't really give you very good feedback.

A better option is to focus your goal on specific actions you can take that will help you achieve your overall objective. For example, if you want to improve your relationship, your goal might be to practise the "four small steps to a better relationship" every day. This is something that you can easily measure.

Even though measurable goals are very important, I think it is equally important to remember your original objective. Otherwise, it is easy to lose yourself in your goals and forget the reason you set them in the first place.

Motivational - Goals need to be motivational. They need to inspire you to take action and make progress. One of the best ways to make goals motivational is to ask yourself why you want to achieve it.

Methodical - Methodical means that you need to think about a strategy for how you are going to accomplish your goal. You don't need to know all the details at first, just start with a general plan.

Meaningful - Your goals should be meaningful to you. This just ensures that they are really your goals, rather than your parent's goals, or society's goals.

Action-Oriented - This means your goal should focus on actions you can take that are in your direct control. It's OK to have goals whose outcome you can't directly control, as long as you are clear about the actions you need to take to do your part in the process.

Achievable - This means that the goal should be achievable. It doesn't mean easy, just that you can have a reasonable expectation of achieving it.

For short-term targets, your probability of achieving the goal should be 80%. Longer term targets could be more of a stretch and have less probability of success.

For your five to ten year vision, you can go for something really big, even if you currently have no idea how to accomplish it.

Realistic - Realistic is another word for achievable. Again, this doesn't mean that the goal needs to be easy. Realistic also means that the actions associated with your goal are things that you can do. For example, if your goal requires you to spend 3 hours at the gym each day, that may not be a very realistic assumption given your present situation and lifestyle.

Relevant - Good goals are relevant to you and to your life. Relevant goals are meaningful and significant; they can make a difference in your life. If a goal is not relevant to you, then you need to ask yourself why you are even contemplating it.

Time-Bound - For goals that have a natural ending (like outcome goals), establishing a clear deadline for them adds an element of urgency and motivation.

Trackable - All goals should be trackable so you can see what your progress is, either in terms of results you are experiencing, or actions you are taking. Tracking your goals helps you determine if you are going in the right direction and make any necessary adjustments along the way.

The best SMART goals are focused, specific, short-term targets that involve things that are under your direct control. This is what makes goals such powerful achievement tools, but it is also what can limit them.

When to use SMART Goals

If you only use SMART goals, you run the risk of losing sight of the big picture, the reasons why you are setting goals in the first place. SMART goals can help you climb the ladder of success step-by-step, only to find that it is leaning against the wrong wall!

That's why you also need longer-term dreams/goals that may not be SMART, but that give you overall direction, motivation, and guidance.

It's when you combine these two types of goals that you can really make tremendous progress.

The Power of Goal Setting

Goal setting is a powerful process for thinking about

your ideal future, and for motivating yourself to turn this vision of the future into reality.

The process of setting goals helps you choose where you want to go in life. By knowing precisely what you want to achieve, you know where you have to concentrate your efforts. You'll also quickly spot the distraction that would otherwise lure you from your course.

Achieving More with Focus

Goal setting techniques are used by top-level athletes, successful business-people and achievers in all fields. They give you long-term vision and short-term motivation. They focus your acquisition of knowledge and help you to organise your time and your resources so that you can make the very most of your life.

By setting sharp, clearly defined goals, you can measure and take pride in the achievement of those goals. You can see forward progress in what might previously have seemed a long pointless grind. By setting goals, you will also raise your self-confidence, as you recognise your ability and competence in achieving the goals that you have set.

Starting to Set Personal Goals

Goals are set on a number of different levels: First you create your "big picture" of what you want to do with your life, and decide what large-scale goals you want to achieve. Second, you break these down into the smaller and smaller targets that you must hit so that you reach your lifetime goals. Finally, once you have your plan, you start working to achieve it.

We start this process with your Lifetime Goals, and work down to the things you can do today to start moving towards them.

Your Lifetime Goals

The first step in setting personal goals is to consider what you want to achieve in your lifetime (or by a time at least, say, ten years in the future) as setting Lifetime Goals gives you the overall perspective that shapes all other aspects of your decision-making.

To give a broad, balanced coverage of all important areas in your life, try to set goals in some of these categories (or in categories of your own, where these are important to you):

✓ **Artistic**
Do you want to achieve any artistic goals? If so, what?

✓ **Attitude**
Is any part of your mindset holding you back? Is there any part of the way that you behave that upsets you? If so, set a goal to improve your behaviour or find a solution to the problem.

✓ **Career**
What level do you want to reach in your career?

✓ Education
Is there any knowledge you want to acquire in particular? What information and skills will you need to achieve other goals?

✓ Family
How do you want to be seen by a partner or by members of your extended family?

✓ Financial
How much do you want to earn?

✓ Physical
Are there any athletic goals you want to achieve, or do you want good health deep into old age? What steps are you going to take to achieve this?

✓ Pleasure
How do you want to enjoy yourself? Is there enough you time in your life for things that you enjoy?

✓ Public Service
Do you want to make the world a better place? Is there a charity you would like to support?

I read somewhere that James Joyce (who wrote *Ulysses)* had a goal about materialism – *Spend a third, save a third, give a third away* – I rather like that sentiment.

So anyway back to the plot, do spend some time on these, and then select one goal in each category that best reflects what you want to do. Then consider trimming again so that you have a small number of really significant goals on which you can focus.

As you do this, make sure that the goals that you have set are ones that you genuinely want to achieve, not ones that your parents, family, or employers might want. (If you have a partner, you probably want to consider what he or she wants, however make sure you also remain true to yourself).

Starting to Achieve Your Lifetime Goals

Once you have set your lifetime goals, set a twenty five year plan of smaller goals that you should complete if you are to reach your lifetime plan. Then set a five year plan, one year plan, six month plan, and one month plan of progressively smaller goals that you should reach to achieve your lifetime goals. Each of these should be based on the previous plan.

Then create a list of things that you should do today to work towards your lifetime goals. At an early stage these goals may be to read books and gather information on the achievement of your goals. This will help you to improve the quality and realism of your goal setting.

Finally review your plans, and make sure that they fit the way in which you want to live your life.

Staying on Course

Once you have decided your first set of plans, keep

the process going by reviewing and updating your to-do list on a daily basis. Periodically review the longer term plans, and modify them to reflect your changing priorities and experience.

Achieving Goals

When you have achieved a goal, take the time to enjoy the satisfaction of having done so. Absorb the implications of the goal achievement, and observe the progress you have made towards other goals. If the goal was a significant one, reward yourself appropriately. All of this helps you build the life you deserve!

With the experience of having achieved this goal, review the rest of your goal plans:

- If you achieved the goal too easily, make your next goals harder.
- If the goal took a dispiriting length of time to achieve, make the next goals a little easier.
- If you learned something that would lead you to change other goals, do so.
- If you noticed a deficit in your skills despite achieving the goal, decide whether to set goals to fix this.

Failure to meet goals does not matter much, as long as you learn from it. Feed lessons learned back into your goal setting programme.

Remember too that your goals will change as time goes on. Adjust them regularly to reflect growth in your knowledge and experience, and if goals do not hold any attraction any longer, then let them go.

Key Points

Goal setting is an important method of:

- Deciding what is important for you to achieve in your life.
- Separating what is important from what is irrelevant, or a distraction.
- Motivating yourself.
- Building your self-confidence, based on successful achievement of goals.

If you don't already set goals, do so, starting now. As you make this technique part of your life, you'll find your career accelerating, and you'll wonder how you did without it!

In the western business world, it is now quite common for employees to take a more active role with their manager in creating their own personal and career development plans. When I first encountered this many years ago, the emphasis was more on my training and development. It did not really involve setting a work goal of any consequence. Empowering individuals in the workplace to become more accountable is now regarded as an essential motivator.

Even though much organisational training and development expertise goes into setting up and maintaining employee career development and performance review programmes, the onus is still fairly and squarely on you to figure out how to make optimal use of them. What frequently happens is that employees leave everything until they get a warning reminder email from their manager; and they then rush to enter goals and objectives into the system before some looming cut-off date.

This is a recipe for disaster because, in their haste, they will be tempted to enter poorly thought-out goals in order to meet the deadline. Or even worse, to add too many goals in order to somehow impress the various managers who hold the promotion, salary or bonus keys. And remember, the unwritten secret of all corporate performance review systems is that 50% of the essential goals, projects and effort that actually arise in any given year will not be on anyone's radar at the start of the year - simply because they haven't come into existence yet. So it is definitely in the employee's best interests to have a minimum number of concise goals, rather than a mishmash of weakly conceived ones.

What if you understand the message in the preceding paragraph but still struggle in coming up with appropriate work goals? The key word here is probably "alignment". Whatever goals you create should be in alignment with both your own vision of your career and life, and also with that of the organisation itself. If you're fortunate, your company will be one that has clear and well communicated statements of what it is about, all the way from boardroom down to divisional and perhaps also departmental level. Should that not be the case then you will need to do some discrete investigations of what is expected from you - perhaps from other departmental managers who do know what is going on.

Let's say you have created your work goals and they're pretty much in alignment with both the company's vision and your own vision of where you want to be and what you want to be doing. And you have supportive management! What then?

Well, here lies another potential trap. Because people are so busy with the 50% of urgent and important projects that are invariably rarely on anyone's agenda or planning tool, you might be tempted to conclude that there just isn't time to focus on career development objectives whose deadlines are at the end of the year; and where the next performance review with your manager is at least six months away!

Such thinking is defeatist and, over time, may habitually condition you to focus exclusively on the "urgent and important", at the expense of the "not urgent but important" goals that typically are on career development programmes.

The solution to this dilemma is to break down the career development goals into the smallest elements you can think of. Then at least once a day spend five to ten minutes on moving the goals forward. For example, if the work goal is to complete an external quality assurance certification which would advance your own career prospects and also be of benefit in building trust with customers, then even though there is an enormous amount of work to be done in order to actually get certified, your very first step may be to find the telephone number of a company which provides appropriate training to help you. Or perhaps it's to get the list of books you need to study into the Finance Department's procurement system for management approval and sign-off.

These numerous five-minute steps will add up over time (certainly after six months) and, if you keep electronic or paper folder records of all the proactive steps you have taken to move forward on the work goal, then your next midyear review with your manager is likely to be more enjoyable, rewarding and productive.

Indeed, goal setting works and it works wonders if you know how to make use of it. Unfortunately, most people who set their goals still fail to achieve them. Why is this so? It is not that they do not know what they want and it is not because they do not know how to set their goal. It is because they do not do what is necessary after they have set their goal.

In fact, it is what you do after you set your goals that will determine your success. Even if you set the most interesting goal in your life, you will never achieve it if you are not doing anything right after you set your goal. These are the three actions you must take right after you set your goal:

- Share your goal with someone close with you. Tell your goal to your family members, your close friends who will support you and tell your loved ones about your goal. You know very well that, the moment you share your dreams with other people, you are putting commitment into them and you will have no other choice but to achieve them.
- Visualise and affirm your goal every morning right after you wake up and right before you sleep. Many people fail to do this because they think that this does not work. If you do this, you will activate the law of attraction and you will motivate yourself by visualising the achievement of your goals. Write down your affirmation on a piece of paper and put it beside your bed so that you can read through and visualise your goal before you sleep and after you wake up.
- Finally, you will never achieve your goal if you are not doing anything about it. Take at least 3 action steps each and every day to make sure that you move closer toward what you want in your life. Many people procrastinate and delay their action and that is why they fail to achieve what they want. If you are serious in making your dreams come true, you must take consistent action every day.

These are the three actions you must take right after you set your goal. Remember, it is what you do after you set your target that will determine your success. It is all about getting things done. As long as you take the necessary action, you will receive results.

It is so easy to give up sometimes; however,

persistence is closely linked with discipline and one feeds off and supports the other in accomplishing your goals.

The classic speech that Winston Churchill made on 29 October 1941 to the boys at Harrow School. *"Never, never, in nothing great or small, large or petty, never give in except to convictions of honour and good sense. Never yield to force; never yield to the apparently overwhelming might of the enemy."*

This certainly encapsulates the determination required in challenging times. There is another factor which is related to both persistence and discipline and which may surprise you. The degree that you have to force yourself to keep to your "discipline" will be to the degree that you are missing a true vision and purpose for what you are doing.

When you have the big picture in mind and have your real area of life passion nailed down, you can work for hours and hours at times without really getting tired or disinterested.

You can get "lost" in your work and wonder where the time went.

In this scenario, discipline becomes easier and if you are finding that you really have to put a lot of effort into persisting and "keeping yourself disciplined", perhaps you need to review your vision (dream) and goals and make sure you really have them nailed down.

That aside, persistence is *the* most important quality that will allow you to stick to your vision, reach your goals and learn what you need to learn to get there and to eventually arrive at your envisioned future.

And of course your paradigm tends to shift as you are moving closer to your goals! These paradigm shifts and "aha" moments are what we live for. They bring us closer to our innermost selves.

People who accomplish their goals did not "have it all worked out" at the beginning and were not always destined to be successful. Some of the greatest failures have transpired within the same people who went on to achieve the greatest successes. Thomas Edison, as we have already pointed out, had tenacity for sure.

Persistence and determination (not luck, parental lineage or even education) are what keep you going when you are having a rough time and want to wander off the path for a few weeks. These are what keep you going in times of confusion or when things are not going the way you want.

But underlying your persistent drive is knowing what your dream or goal is in the first place and really *wanting* it. Without that, you have nothing to persist toward.

> *Man is a goal seeking animal. His life only has meaning if he is reaching out and striving for his goals.*
>
> —*Aristotle*

How to Work Wonders with Personal Goals

- ✓ Embrace the benefits of what you want to achieve.
- ✓ Set goals that are personal to you and that you are committed to.
- ✓ Know exactly what it is you want to achieve.
- ✓ Know how to measure your goals.
- ✓ Ensure that your goals are achievable.
- ✓ Write your goals down – *very important.*
- ✓ Make sure that you set timelines.
- ✓ Design a visionary board.
- ✓ Use visualisation.
- ✓ Use positive affirmations.
- ✓ Believe in yourself.
- ✓ Stickability – Don't give up.
- ✓ Share your plans with others and ask for support.
- ✓ Learn from your mistakes.
- ✓ Reward yourself for every achievement.
- ✓ Don't give up.

Work Wonders at Home

The role of the traditional office is changing rapidly as employers and staff increasingly look to adopt smarter ways of working.

The *2007 Flexible Working Survey*, compiled by facilities management firm *Johnson Controls,* shows that employers are using a mixed approach to how and where staff work.

Rather than completely abandoning the traditional corporate office, the research shows that employees are using a mix of home, remote and office working as part of a combined package.

More than 60% of the staff questioned said they used a combination of office, home and remote working, while 35% said it was not important to go into the office at all.

The research shows that flexible working has become far more main stream in the past five years, with staff spending more time hot-desking, working from home, or working remotely.

Here are a few tips that can help you if you find yourself working from home

✓ Get yourself ready, just as if you were going to an office. If you feel like a professional, you'll work like one.
✓ Start the day with a clear purpose. Know what your most important tasks are.
✓ Set a time frame for projects/activities and keep to it work.
✓ Find your best hours for working - high energy, low interruptions.
✓ Take breaks in between tasks. Go for a short walk, get a drink of water.
✓ Let your family know that certain times are for work, and you can't be disturbed for non-emergencies.
✓ Fit a trip to the shops into your lunch break.
✓ Do not do your home chores in work allocated time.
✓ Set yourself office hours.
✓ Invest in the right tools and technology.
✓ A good-sized desk and quality chair.
✓ Develop a back-up plan in case there is a hardware or internet problem, back up your hard drive regularly, know where you can get internet access if it fails at home.
✓ Take pride in your space. Your work area should be clean, with good light and air circulation.
✓ A closed door to your office is an under-appreciated asset when you have small children and pets especially if taking business calls.

✓ Communicate the boundaries of your space and time to your family.

Sometimes when you work from home you can feel quite isolated. If you feel lonely and need some human interaction, here are a few suggestions for social contact.

✓ Go out for lunch with others.
✓ Go to the gym at lunchtime and do a work out.
✓ Go and work at the local "Green Tea" shop for a few hours.
✓ Have a work friend who works from home too who you can call for support or to bounce ideas.

The concept of working from home and having flexibility in working hours can be a great advantage to work/life balance, it can also work the other way if you do not separate the two. Good planning, organisation and self discipline is the key to making it work well for you.

Summary

This book provides you with a selection box of ideas to help you to improve your workplace wellness as well as many tips and advice that will help you in your personal life.

Sometimes when you are feeling discouraged at work, I suggest you start reading about positive motivational quotes to encourage and empower yourself. You will start feeling better in yourself.

How to Work Wonders – Top Tips

✓ Refuse the snooze on your alarm.
✓ Start the day with hot water and lemon.
✓ Set yourself a priority action plan.
✓ Thoughts feed emotion – think positively.
✓ Keep a bottle of water with you.
✓ Wear a pedometer to work.
✓ Avoid refined carbohydrates and sugar.
✓ Avoid excess caffeine.
✓ Introduce walking meetings.
✓ Read inspirational quotes.
✓ Use SUMO – shut up and move on!.
✓ Look after your environment.

Motivational Quotations

Here is a select compilation of positive quotes about work to inspire you:

Aristotle
Pleasure in the job puts perfection in the work.

Catherine Pulsifer
Remember that you are needed. There is at least one important work to be done that will not be done unless you do it.

Theodore Roosevelt
Do what you can, with what you have, where you are.

Mahatma Gandhi
A man is the sum of his actions, of what he has done, of what he can do, Nothing else.

Theodore Roosevelt
Far and away the best prize that life has to offer is the chance to work hard at work worth doing.

James M. Barrie
Nothing is really work unless you would rather be doing something else.

Ralph Waldo Emerson
The reward of a thing well done is to have done it.

Dale Carnegie
Criticism of others is futile and if you indulge in it often you should be warned that it can be fatal to your career.

Bobby Unser
Desire! That's the one secret of every man's career. Not education. Not being born with hidden talents. Desire.

Brian Tracy
If you wish to achieve worthwhile things in your personal and career life, you must become a worthwhile person in your own self-development.

Lou Holtz
I think everyone should experience defeat at least once during their career. You learn a lot from it.

Mark Twain
Keep away from people who try to belittle your ambitions. Small people always do that, but the really great make you feel that you, too, can become great.

Hamilton Holt
Nothing worthwhile comes easily. Work, continuous work and hard work, is the only way to accomplish results that last.

Napoleon Hill
When defeat comes, accept it as a signal that your plans are not sound, rebuild those plans, and set sail once more toward your coveted goal.

Brian Tracy
Only undertake what you can do in an excellent fashion. There are no prizes for average performance.

Indira Gandhi
There are two kinds of people, those who do the work and those who take the credit. Try to be in the first group; there is less competition there.

Henry L. Doherty
Plenty of men can do good work for a spurt and with immediate promotion in mind, but for promotion you want a man in whom good work has become a habit.

A Creed for Life - *Desiderata*

*Go placidly amid the noise and the haste,
and remember what peace there may be in silence.*
***

*As far as possible, without surrender,
be on good terms with all persons.
Speak your truth quietly and clearly;
and listen to others,
even to the dull and the ignorant;
they too have their story.
Avoid loud and aggressive persons;
they are vexatious to the spirit.*
***

*If you compare yourself with others,
you may become vain or bitter,
for always there will be greater and lesser persons
than yourself.
Enjoy your achievements as well as your plans.
Keep interested in your own career, however humble;
it is a real possession in the changing fortunes of time.*
***

*Exercise caution in your business affairs,
for the world is full of trickery.
But let this not blind you to what virtue there is;
many persons strive for high ideals,
and everywhere life is full of heroism.*

Be yourself. Especially do not feign affection.
Neither be cynical about love,
for in the face of all aridity and disenchantment,
it is as perennial as the grass.
***

Take kindly the counsel of the years,
gracefully surrendering the things of youth.
Nurture strength of spirit to shield you in sudden
misfortune.
But do not distress yourself with dark imaginings.
Many fears are born of fatigue and loneliness.
***

Beyond a wholesome discipline,
be gentle with yourself.
You are a child of the universe
no less than the trees and the stars;
you have a right to be here.
And whether or not it is clear to you,
no doubt the universe is unfolding as it should.
***

Therefore be at peace with God,
whatever you conceive Him to be.
And whatever your labors and aspirations,
in the noisy confusion of life,
keep peace in your soul.
***

With all its sham, drudgery, and broken dreams,
it is still a beautiful world.
Be cheerful. Strive to be happy.

Workplace Wellness

Workplace Wellness is a recognised programme that is delivered in organisations as a bite size half day learning activity by a range of accredited professionals. With a practical interactive approach it provides a great opportunity for organisations to raise awareness for their staff.

For more information by email contact info@thelearningarchitect.com

or call 00044 (0) 1242 700027 for more details.

Motivational Speaking

Liggy Webb is a keynote motivational speaker and a leading expert in the area of *Workplace Wellness* and *Personal Excellence.*

If you would like Liggy to speak at one of your events please contact us by emailing info@thelearning architect.com or phone 0044 (0) 1242 700027.

The Learning Architect

The Learning Architect is an exciting and diverse people development organisation that works with key industry professionals who are experts in their niche field and who have amassed a high level of professional knowledge. Key services include:

- **Workplace Wellness** - The mental, physical and environmental health of people is now the number one priority for many organisations. We offer a range of organisational staff surveys, bespoke learning programmes, bite size workshops, motivational speaking and *Workplace Wellness* materials.
- **Motivational Speaking** - Key note motivational speaking at staff conferences and away days are becoming an increasingly popular way to motivate and inspire people. We provide expert industry specialists who will speak on a variety of topical issues that will add value and spice to your event.
- **Leadership Development** - We help leaders to 'look in the mirror' at their personal performance, define areas for improvement and develop them in context of the business challenges they face. We develop leaders by changing their behaviour and developing their capabilities.
- **Management Development** - We help managers learn and improve their skills and offer a range of programmes including: Performance Management , Communication Skills, Appraisal Skills, Change Management, Coaching and Mentoring, Counselling Skills, Stress Management and Time Management.

- **Sales Development -** We can help you to develop your business and your people in a variety of ways using solutions including: Consultative Selling, Sales Process Management, Marketing, Negotiation, Presentation Skills, Business Networking and Exhibition Excellence all tailored to suit the needs of your business.
- **Personal Development -** Employees need to take responsibility for their own professional development to improve areas where they lack skills. We offer a range of solutions including: Time Management, Assertiveness Skills, Conflict Management, Personal and Emotional Intelligence.
- **Team Development -** The Learning Architect team development experts can design and deliver a range of solutions to fully meet the needs of your organisation. Connecting people to each other helps to establish high performing teams and improves general communication and workplace dynamics.
- **Forum Theatre** - We are a leading exponent of the powerful training process called Forum Theatre which won a 2007 National Training Award under the delivery of Tim Stockil. By using actors and audience interaction we can bring alive a variety of topics to fully engage people within organisations.
- **Online Learning Tools -** We offer a variety of online learning tools including the very popular Facet 5 psychometric .We also offer bespoke e learning programmes as an integrated approach to support and supplement some of our key learning areas.

The Learning Architect can provide a range of case studies – For more details please contact us on info@thelearningarchitect.com.

www.thelearningarchitect.com

The Chrysalis Programme

Just imagine a development programme that engages, inspires and compels offenders to make a sustainable change in their lives! A development programme that fits with end-to-end offender management ensuring that offenders are provided the best possible opportunity to change their offending behaviours.

The Learning Architect works in collaboration with the Chrysalis Programme which combines leading-edge people transformational and behavioural development of the calibre that would normally only be made available to senior executives. The content has been adjusted specifically for the audience.

The Chrysalis Programme is a personal leadership and effectiveness development programme that is being applied to offender client groups. The Learning Architect provides tailored Wellness modules and specialist consultants to assist this Programme.

The Chrysalis Programme taps into proven corporate development programmes, resources and expertise, then combines it with best practice from *Offender Management Services*, Mentoring and 'real' work placements to create a fresh approach to offender development and rehabilitation. All this integrates with community sentencing requirements into a single holistic development programme delivered over 12 modules, the culmination of which leads to a level 2 BTEC work skills qualification for the participants.

The Chrysalis Programme has been developed with input, support and/or endorsements from: Lord Ouseley, Dean Ayling SW England Probation Service, HMP Reading, Deirdre Newham - Chair of Northampton Police Authority/Magistrate, Dr Stephen Covey and Dr Edward De-Bono and many of the leading experts in development and behavioural change, to name just a few of our contributors/supporters.

We believe that creating confidence and capability in individuals is key to harnessing their latent potential to develop and grow, because:

There is nothing about a caterpillar that tells you it's going to be a butterfly

The Chrysalis Programme is centrally funded and so is either subsidised or fully funded (free at point of use) for those working with offenders.

For more information contact info@thelearningarchitect.com.

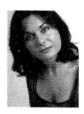

About the Author

Liggy Webb is based in Cheltenham and is the founder director of *The Learning Architect* an international people development organisation. As an experienced *learning and development* professional she works as a consultant with a wide range of organisations including the *United Nations* and the *NHS.*

Through extensive research she has developed a unique holistic approach to personal and professional wellness and is invited to speak on the subject across the world.

Liggy is commited to raising awareness and support for mental health and is involved with a range of key initiatives.

Her next book *H.A.P.P.Y* is out later in the year and is a guide to personal happiness and wellbeing.

For any feedback or information

Please contact liggy@thelearningarchitect.com